ULTRASOUND FOR THE WIN!

EMERGENCY DEPARTMENT CASES

VOLUME 1

JEFFREY SHIH, MD, RDMS

MICHELLE LIN, MD

First Edition, September 2016

ISBN: 978-0-9907948-6-8

www.jshihmd.com

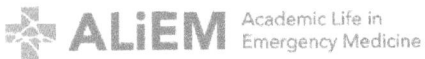

ALiEM Academic Life in
Emergency Medicine

ISBN 9780990794868

9 780990 794868

90000 >

TABLE OF CONTENTS

ABOUT THE AUTHORS

Dr. Jeffrey Shih completed an Emergency Medicine Residency at the Mayo Clinic in Rochester, Minnesota, and an Emergency Ultrasound Fellowship at Yale University in New Haven, Connecticut. He is currently practicing Emergency Medicine in Toronto, Canada, is a Lecturer at University of Toronto, and Program Director of the Emergency Ultrasound Fellowship Program at The Scarborough Hospital.

@jshihmd

Dr. Michelle Lin completed an Emergency Medicine Residency at Harbor-UCLA in Torrance, California. She is the Founder and Chief Executive Officer of Academic Life in Emergency Medicine (ALiEM), a blog-based health professions education innovation organization. She is also a Professor of Emergency Medicine at the University of California, San Francisco Department of Emergency Medicine.

@m_lin

LIST OF CONTRIBUTORS

Rob Bryant, MD
Assistant Professor
Division of Emergency Medicine
University of Utah School of Medicine

Kristin Carmody, MD
Assistant Professor, Co-Director, Emergency Ultrasound Fellowship
Department of Emergency Medicine
NYU Langone Medical Center/Bellevue Hospital Center

EC "Drake" Coffey, MD
Assistant Professor
Department of Emergency Medicine
University of Texas Health Science Center San Antonio

M. Kennedy Hall, MD, MHS
Acting Instructor
Department of Emergency Medicine
University of Washington School of Medicine

Tobias Kummer, MD
Assistant Professor
Department of Emergency Medicine
Mayo Clinic College of Medicine

Stephen Leech, MD
Ultrasound Director, Graduate Medical Education
Department of Emergency Medicine
Orlando Health

Resa E. Lewiss, MD
Director of Point-of-Care Ultrasound
Department of Emergency Medicine
University of Colorado School of Medicine

Mike Mallin, MD
Associate Professor
Division of Emergency Medicine
University of Utah School of Medicine

Christopher L. Moore, MD
Associate Professor
Yale University School of Medicine
Department of Emergency Medicine

Arun Nagdev, MD
Director, Emergency Ultrasound
Department of Emergency Medicine
Highland General Hospital

Mike Stone, MD
Emergency Physician
Department of Emergency Medicine
Legacy Emanuel Medical Center

PREFACE

Since it's inception in the medical field in the early 1960s, the use of ultrasound to aid in the diagnosis of pathology has been steadily increasing. Today, the vast use of ultrasound is becoming increasingly more common-place in medicine, with the training of residents and even medical students, mid-level providers, and prehospital personnel as an aid with procedures and providing a safer standard of patient care.

The Emergency Physician's (EP) role of examining and treating a patient with often limited information and weeding out the "sick" from the "not sick" in a time-sensitive and chaotic environment is ripe for the use of bedside ultrasonography. The opportunity to "cheat" and look at a patient's heart, aorta, gallbladder, or tens of other organs right at the bedside, provides EPs and other emergency providers the ability to better and more accurately diagnose and treat their patients.

The following cases* presented in this book are based on real-life scenarios encountered by EPs who, with the skills and knowledge of Emergency Ultrasonography were able to make quick diagnoses that altered the management and course of a patient's treatment. These ultrasound "saves" highlight the usefulness of bedside ultrasonography in the daily practice of EPs.

While many cases involve the use of advanced ultrasound techniques, they are all readily learnable and are performed by EPs and other healthcare providers. This book should not be used to supplement a formal course in the training of emergency ultrasound. An understanding and familiarity with the basic concepts of bedside ultrasound is assumed of the reader. This collection of cases should be used to learn new ways of using ultrasound in your daily practice, new techniques that can be learned, and to highlight the power of point-of-care ultrasound to provide better, faster, and more patient-centered care.

I hope that through these cases, you can learn and realize the many different ways in which Emergency Providers are using bedside ultrasound to save lives every single day.

Jeffrey Shih, MD, RDMS
Lecturer, University of Toronto;
Program Director,
Emergency Ultrasound Fellowship Program,
The Scarborough Hospital

*Note: All identifying information and certain aspects of the case have been changed to maintain patient confidentiality and protected health information (PHI).

Acknowledgement: Most cases and ultrasound clips are courtesy of the *Yale University* Emergency Department.

101M with Altered Mental Status

OBJECTIVES

1. Determine a broad differential diagnosis of an elderly patient presenting with hypotension and altered mental status
2. Understand the role of point-of-care ultrasound in narrowing the differential diagnosis
3. Recognize the sonographic landmarks utilized in the identification of the abdominal aorta
4. Learn the proper measurement technique and diagnostic criteria for an abdominal aortic aneurysm (AAA)
5. Understand the utility, role, and limitations of point-of-care ultrasound in the identification of a AAA

CASE PRESENTATION

A 101-year-old man with hypertension is brought to the Emergency Department (ED) by ambulance after family members found him down at his home. Paramedics obtained an initial blood pressure of 63/39, which improved to 114/68 after a 1-liter bolus of intravenous fluids. Upon arrival in the ED, he is confused and unable to provide a reliable history. Physical examination reveals a pale and diaphoretic elderly man with no obvious signs of trauma. There are no palpable masses on abdominal examination. He complains only of back pain while the physical examination is being performed.

VITAL SIGNS

BP	89/68 mmHg
P	86 bpm
RR	20 breaths/min
O2	98% room air
T	37.2°C

DIFFERENTIAL DIAGNOSIS

Abdominal aortic aneurysm
Acute coronary syndrome
Aortic dissection
Infection
Metabolic abnormality
Stroke
Syncope
Toxidrome/overdose
Traumatic injury

INITIAL WORKUP

Given the broad differential diagnosis of an altered and hypotensive elderly patient with no reliable history, blood work was drawn and the emergency physician performed a point-of-care ultrasound given his hemodynamic instability and complaint of back pain.

POINT-OF-CARE ULTRASOUND was performed which showed the following:

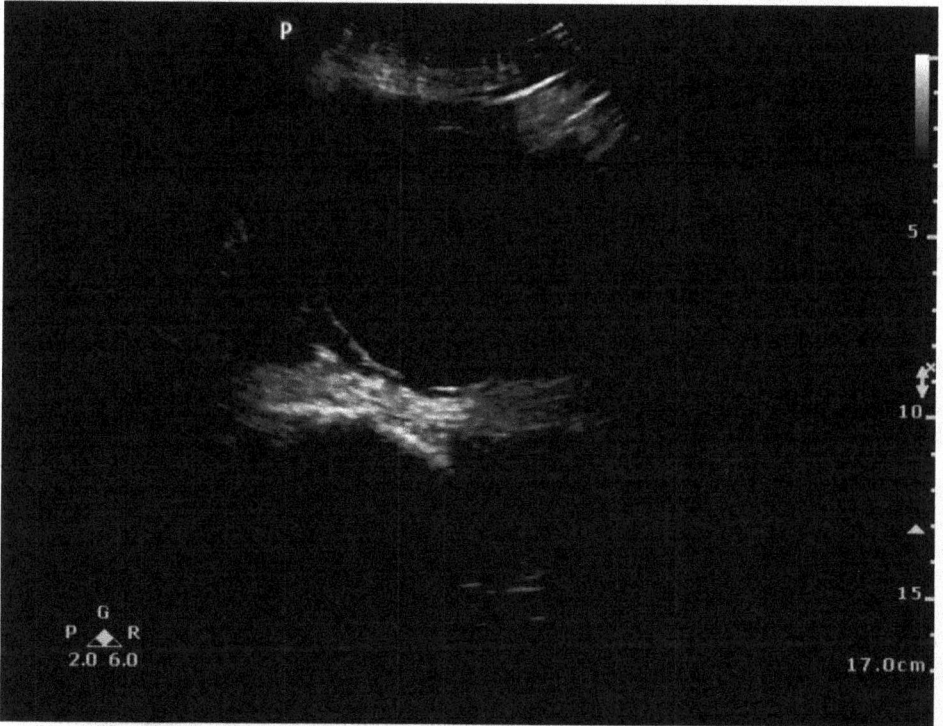

Figure 1.1

Abdominal ultrasound reveals a large 8-9 cm abdominal aortic aneurysm.

The bedside ultrasound shows a large abdominal aortic aneurysm (AAA) (Fig. 1.1), defined as a diameter greater than 3.0 cm, with positive free fluid in Morrison's Pouch (Fig. 1.2, 1.3). Together with the clinical findings, this is highly suspicious for a ruptured AAA. Of note, a FAST may still be negative in the setting of a ruptured AAA with a retroperitoneal hemorrhage.

Figure 1.2

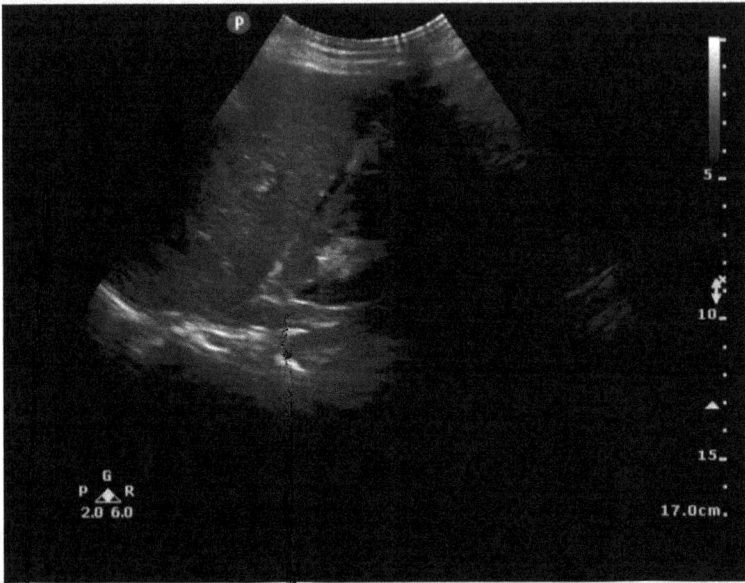

FAST exam reveals the presence of free fluid in Morrison's Pouch

Figure 1.3

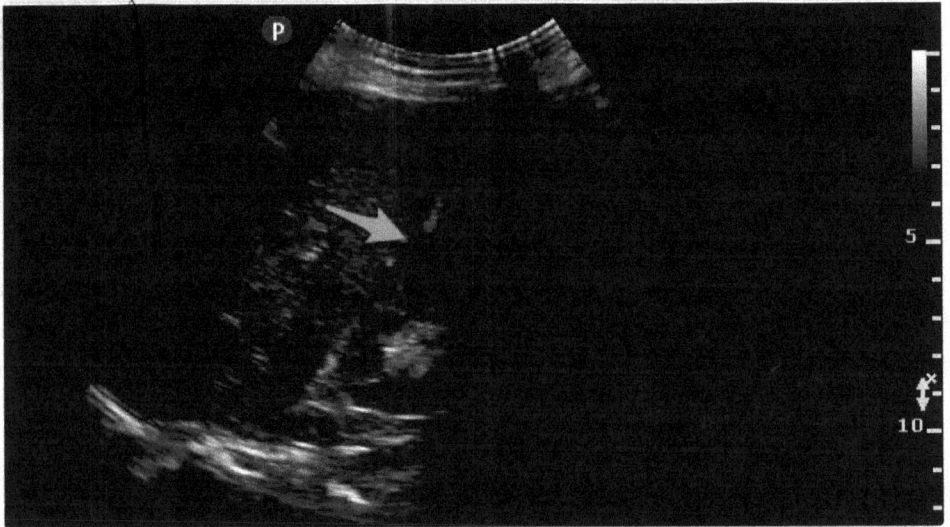

Free fluid (arrow) in Morrison's Pouch

4

ULTRASOUND IMAGE QUALITY ASSURANCE

Point-of-care ultrasonography of the aorta is one of the essential and critical skills that every emergency medicine provider must have. It has the utility of being able to provide a quick and potentially life-saving diagnosis, especially in the patient who is too unstable for computed tomography (CT) scan.

The exam involves using the curvilinear probe, whose low frequency is often necessary to visualize the aorta, especially in obese patients. The abdominal aorta sits anterior to the spine, which provides a convenient sonographic landmark that aids in identification of the aorta. In a transverse orientation, the spine appears as a hyperechoic "horseshoe sign" with posterior shadowing (Fig. 1.4).

Figure 1.4

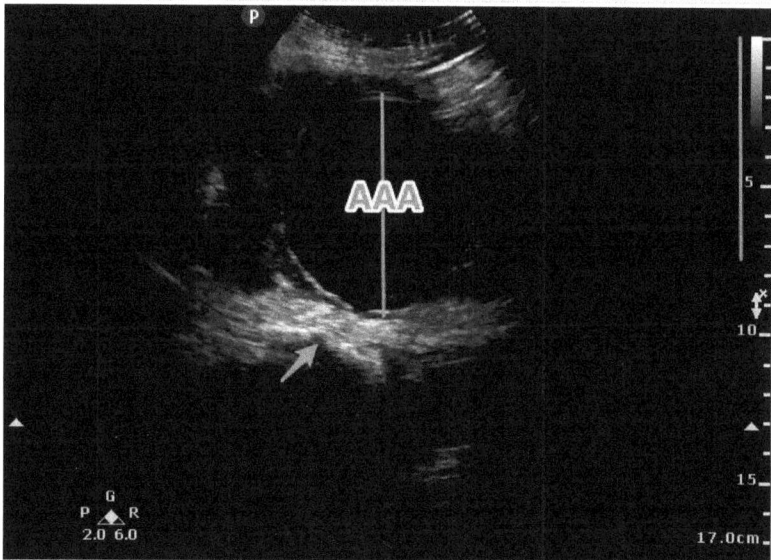

Large abdominal aortic aneurysm (AAA) measured at 7.5 cm, sits just anterior to the spine, the "horseshoe sign" (arrow) with posterior shadowing.

A full examination of the abdominal aorta involves scanning through in a transverse plane starting proximally from the subxiphoid area at the level of the superior mesenteric artery (SMA), and though to the bifurcation at the iliac arteries. A measurement of greater than 3.0 cm, made from the outer wall to outer wall, is considered aneurysmal. Ideally, 3 measurements (proximal, mid, and distal) should be made along the abdominal aorta, including a longitudinal (sagittal) view.

Common pitfalls include the inability to adequately visualize the aorta due to overlying bowel gas, and incorrect measurement. Bowel gas can be gently pushed out of the way by applying firm, steady pressure with the ultrasound probe. Measurement of the abdominal aorta, as mentioned previously, should be measured "outer wall-to-outer wall", to avoid potentially measuring a false lumen of a large AAA with an intramural thrombus (Fig. 1.5).

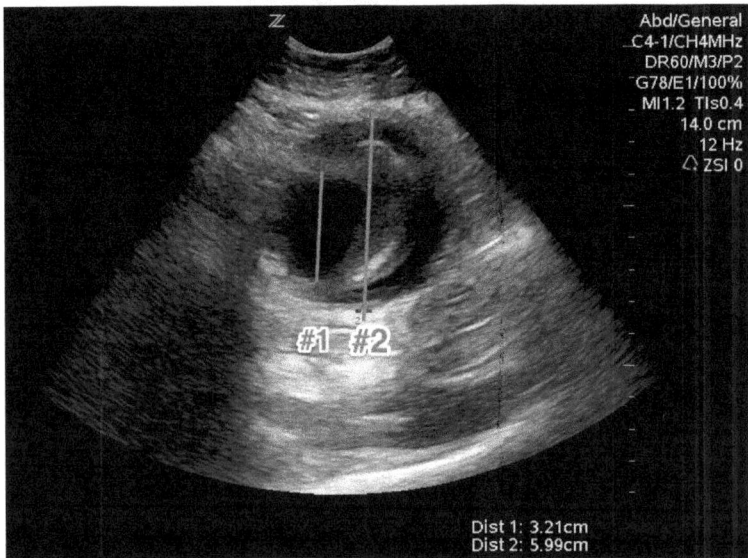

Figure 1.5

Pitfall: Measuring a false pseudo-lumen of a large abdominal aortic aneurysm with an intraluminal clot (#1 - incorrect measurement, #2 - correct measurement).

DISPOSITION AND CASE CONCLUSION

Given the findings on the point-of-care ultrasound (a large AAA with free fluid in Morrison's pouch) in the right clinical setting, the patient had a ruptured AAA until proven otherwise. The massive transfusion protocol was activated, and vascular surgery was emergently consulted.

The decision was made to obtain a stat CT scan to confirm the diagnosis, as he was momentarily hemodynamically stable with aggressive resuscitation. The CT confirmed the findings of a large ruptured AAA (Fig. 1.6).

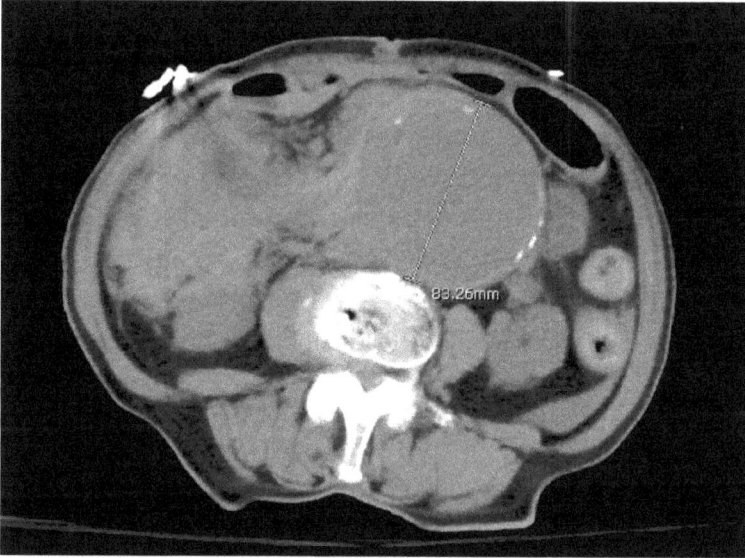

Figure 1.6

83.26mm

CT reveals a large abdominal aortic aneurysm measuring up to 8.5 cm with evidence of high density intraperitoneal fluid consistent with rupture of abdominal aortic aneurysm.

The vascular surgery and emergency medicine teams had a collaborative discussion with the patient's family regarding his poor prognosis and unlikelihood that he would survive surgery. The patient's family ultimately decided to make him comfort care only.

The point-of-care ultrasound in this case was able to quickly identify the patient's diagnosis of a ruptured AAA and vascular surgery was emergently consulted. Unfortunately, due to the high mortality associated with a ruptured AAA and the patient's advanced age, he did not survive. However this doesn't diminish the critical role of bedside ultrasonography in patients at risk for AAA.

An estimated 5% of the population over the age of 50 are estimated to have a AAA, and the incidence of this potentially life-threatening disease in the United States has been increasing over the past few decades [1]. However despite this, more than 80% of patients are unaware of their aneurysmal disease [5]. This makes the diagnosis of a ruptured AAA challenging. Additionally, the presenting symptoms of a ruptured AAA are often non-specific, and patients will often not have hemodynamic instability until there has been significant disease progression and blood loss. The most common misdiagnoses include renal colic, acute diverticulitis, and gastrointestinal bleed.

The physical examination in patients with aortic aneurysms has been studied and found to be unreliable; the ability to palpate a pulsatile mass on physical examination has been shown to detect only 39% of all AAAs [3]. Furthermore, the 'classic triad' of ruptured AAA that is often taught consisting of abdominal or flank pain, palpable abdominal mass, and hypotension has also been proven to be unreliable, and is present in only 30-50% of cases of ruptured AAA [5].

The mortality rate of a ruptured AAA is high at an estimated 90%, with greater than 10,000 deaths annually in the United States [1][2]. The utility of a real-time point-of-care imaging modality like ultrasound is vital to the prompt diagnosis, and has been shown to decrease mortality from 75% to 35% [4].

While CT is considered the gold-standard for diagnosis of AAA, ultrasonography of the aorta by emergency physicians has been shown to have a general agreement compared with radiology-read CT imaging. There have been several studies proving that ultrasonography is accurate, approaching 100% sensitivity and specificity [Table 1.1].

	Sample Size	% Sensitivity (95% CI)	% Specificity (95% CI)
Lanoix et al. 2000	21	100	94.1
Kuhn et al. 2000	68	100	95.2
Rowland et al. 2001	33	100	100
Jones et al. 2003	66	97.5	100
Tayal et al. 2003	125	100	98
Knaut et al. 2005	104	100	97
Costantino et al. 2005	238	94	100

Table 1.1. *Summary of sensitivity and specificity of ultrasound to detect an abdominal aortic aneurysm. Adapted from Rubano et al. 2013 [6]*

When performed early in the workup of a patient suspected of having a ruptured AAA, as was done in this case, bedside ultrasound can expedite surgical consultation and definitive care.

TAKE-HOME POINTS

1. There is an increasing prevalence of AAA in the United States in patients who are unaware of their aneurysmal disease, and a ruptured AAA can be a difficult and elusive diagnosis that is associated with a high mortality rate.

2. Point-of-care ultrasonography is the imaging modality of choice in unstable patients with suspicion for AAA, and can expedite surgical consultation and definitive management.

3. Emergency physicians can correctly identify AAA (defined as >3 cm) on bedside ultrasonography with 94% sensitivity and 100% specificity [7].

REFERENCES

1. Knaut AL, Kendall JL, Patten R, Ray C. Ultrasonographic measurement of aortic diameter by emergency physicians approximates results obtained by computed tomography. J Emerg Med. 2005 Feb;28(2):119-26. PMID: 15707804.

2. Fink HA, Lederle FA, Roth CS, Bowles CA, Nelson DB, Haas MA. The accuracy of physical examination to detect abdominal aortic aneurysm. Arch Intern Med. 2000 Mar 27;160(6):833-6. PMID: 10737283.

3. Lederle FA, Simel DL. The rational clinical examination. Does this patient have abdominal aortic aneurysm?. JAMA. 1999 Jan 6;281(1):77-82. PMID: 9892455.

4. Hoffman M, Avellone JC, Plecha FR, Rhodes RS, Donovan DL, Beven EG, DePalma RG, Frisch JA. Operation for ruptured abdominal aortic aneurysms: a community-wide experience. Surgery. 1982 May;91(5):597-602. PMID: 7071748.

5. Marston WA, Ahlquist R, Johnson G Jr, Meyer AA. Misdiagnosis of ruptured abdominal aortic aneurysms. J Vasc Surg. 1992 Jul;16(1):17-22. PMID: 1619721.

6. Rubano E, Mehta N, Caputo W, Paladino L, Sinert R. Systematic review: emergency department bedside ultrasonography for diagnosing suspected abdominal aortic aneurysm. Acad Emerg Med. 2013 Feb;20(2):128-38. PMID: 23406071.

7. Costantino TG, Bruno EC, Handly N, Dean AJ. Accuracy of emergency medicine ultrasound in the evaluation of abdominal aortic aneurysm. J Emerg Med. 2005 Nov;29(4):455-60. PMID: 16243207.

28F with Shortness of Breath

OBJECTIVES

1. Identify the differences between the cardiology and emergency medicine probe marker orientation conventions.
2. Recognize the direct and indirect echocardiographic findings suggestive of right heart strain and pulmonary embolism (PE).
3. Describe McConnell Sign and its relevance to the diagnosis of PE.

CASE PRESENTATION

A 28-year-old female with active cancer on chemotherapy presents to the ED with 1-week of progressively worsening shortness of breath. On examination, the patient appears distressed, tachypneic, and requires 15L O2 via a non-rebreather face mask to maintain a normal oxygen saturation.

VITAL SIGNS

BP	102/69 mmHg
P	142 bpm
RR	22 breaths/min
O2	100% on 15L oxygen via non-rebreather face mask
T	36.9°C

DIFFERENTIAL DIAGNOSIS

Congestive heart failure

Pericardial effusion

Pleural effusion

Pneumonia

Pneumothorax

Pulmonary embolism

POINT-OF-CARE ULTRASOUND was performed which showed the following:

Figure 2.1

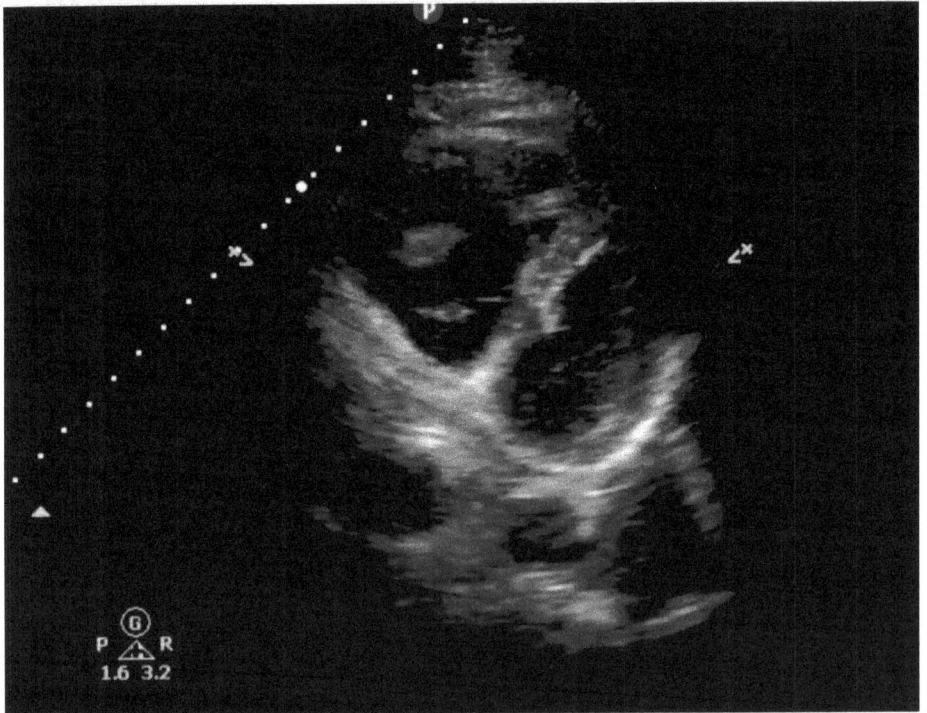

Parasternal view of revealing an intra-ventricular thrombus and dilated right ventricle

Figure 2.2

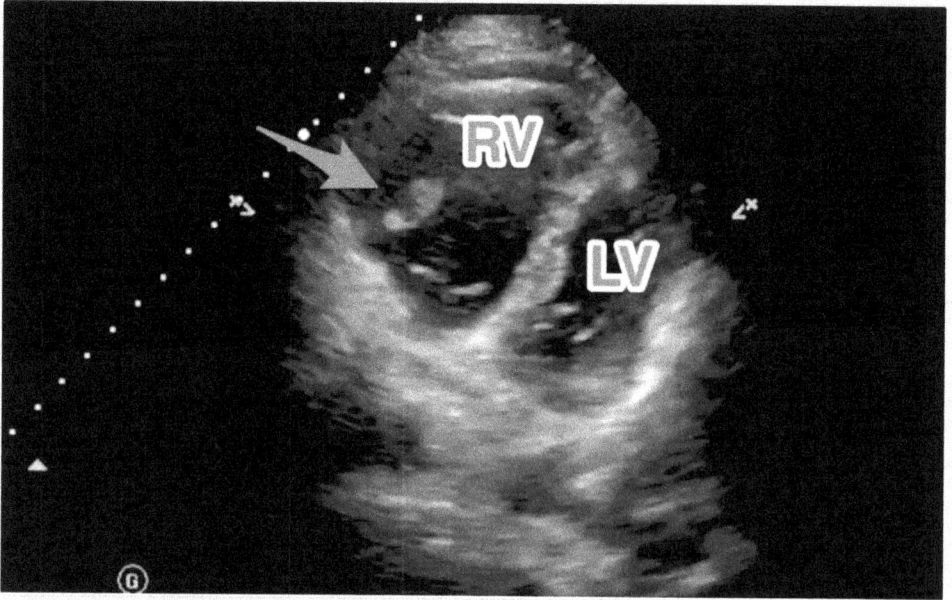

Bedside echocardiogram showing intra-ventricular thrombus (arrow) and dilated right ventricle.
RV = right ventricle; LV = left ventricle

Immediately evident on bedside echocardiogram are distinct ultrasonographic findings that are highly suggestive of a pulmonary embolism (PE):

1. Figure 2.1: Right ventricular hypokinesis with apical sparing (McConnell Sign).

2. Figure 2.2: An intra-ventricular thrombus within a dilated right ventricle (blue arrow), with an RV to LV size ratio greater than 1:1 indicative of right heart strain. Visualization of a clot is a rare (estimated to be present in only 4-18% of acute PE [1]) but specific echocardiographic finding.

In this clinical context, the bedside echocardiogram findings are highly suggestive of an acute PE.

	Echocardiographic Findings in Acute Pulmonary Embolism
Direct	Right heart thrombus
	PA thrombus
Indirect	RV dilation (> 1:1 RV:LV ratio)
	McConnell Sign
	RV dysfunction
	DVT on lower extremity US

Table 2.1. *Direct and indirect echocardiographic findings in acute pulmonary embolism (PA = pulmonary artery; RV = right ventricle; LV = left ventricle DVT = deep vein thrombosis; US = ultrasound)*

ULTRASOUND IMAGE QUALITY ASSURANCE

An important aspect of ultrasonography is appropriate and optimal image acquisition. Figure 2.1 shows an apical view of the heart with appropriate depth and gain. While the providers were not able to obtain an apical 4-chamber view, the right and left ventricles are clearly demonstrated, and the clip is of sufficient quality to provide valuable diagnostic information. Patients with acute respiratory distress can be challenging to image due to tachypnea and the inability to turn to a left lateral decubitus position.

Of note, the probe indicator-to-screen orientation is oriented to the patient's right, which is the reverse of the cardiology convention [2]. Whether you use the ED or cardiology convention, it is important to know how you are oriented so that you are properly identifying the right and left sides of the heart especially when trying to identify pathology such as right heart strain. In this case, the right side of the heart is on the left side of the screen. If the probe is reversed, one can misinterpret a normal LV as being a RV.

The clip could be improved by attempting to better visualize both atria so that all four chambers are in view. In addition, the interventricular septum should be ideally oriented vertically down the screen rather than on an angle as in the clip. Sliding the transducer laterally so that the septum is centered on the screen, and angling the beam back towards the inferior tip of the right scapula will result in a more vertical orientation to the interventricular septum.

DISPOSITION AND CASE CONCLUSION

A CT angiogram of the chest was obtained which revealed a massive PE extending from the RV causing near-total occlusion of bilateral pulmonary arteries extending to all segmental pulmonary arteries. Heparin was started in the ED, and the patient was admitted to the medical intensive care unit. The patient continued to decompensate during her admission, and tPA was administered with subsequent clinical improvement. Ultimately, the patient was discharged home on enoxaparin after a full recovery with normal oxygen saturations.

TAKE-HOME POINTS

1. Bedside echocardiogram, in correlation with the appropriate clinical picture, can be a beneficial diagnostic tool in the unstable patient with suspicion for acute PE.

2. Echocardiographic features of PE can be classified into direct (high specificity, low sensitivity) and indirect (low specificity, moderate sensitivity) findings (Table 2.1) [3].

3. McConnell sign, which is RV hypokinesis with apical sparing, in its original description was found to be 77% sensitive and 94% specific for diagnosing PE [4]. However, more recent literature has shown that McConnell sign is non-specific, found in 2/3 of patients with RV infarction [5], and should not be used in isolation for the diagnosis of PE, nor for the decision to adminster thrombolytics.

4. Be aware of the differences between the ED and cardiology echo conventions to avoid confusion and potential misinterpretation of findings.

REFERENCES

1. Sökmen G, Sökmen A, Yasim A, Oksüz H. Witnessed migration of a giant, free-floating thrombus into the right atrium during echocardiography, leading to fatal pulmonary embolism. Turk Kardiyol Dern Ars. 2009 Jan;37(1):41-3. PMID: 19225252.

2. Moore C. Current issues with emergency cardiac ultrasound probe and image conventions. Acad Emerg Med. 2008 Mar;15(3):278-84. PMID: 18304059.

3. Borloz MP, Frohna WJ, Phillips CA, Antonis MS. Emergency department focused bedside echocardiography in massive pulmonary embolism. J Emerg Med. 2011 Dec;41(6):658-60. PMID: 21820258.

4. McConnell MV, Solomon SD, Rayan ME, Come PC, Goldhaber SZ, Lee RT. Regional right ventricular dysfunction detected by echocardiography in acute pulmonary embolism. Am J Cardiol. 1996 Aug 15;78(4):469-73. PMID: 8752195.

5. Casazza F, Bongarzoni A, Capozi A, Agostoni O. Regional right ventricular dysfunction in acute pulmonary embolism and right ventricular infarction. Eur J Echocardiogr. 2005 Jan;6(1):11-4. PMID: 15664548.

93F with Chest Pain

OBJECTIVES

1. Describe the utility of point-of-care ultrasound in the identification of thoracic aortic aneurysms (TAA).
2. Identify the ideal echocardiographic window when attempting to visualize and measure the aortic root.
3. Know the normal measurement of the thoracic aortic root and what measurement determines an aneurysm.

CASE PRESENTATION

A 93-year-old female with no available medical history is brought to the Emergency Department by ambulance after she was noted to clutch her chest and collapse while at home. She is unable to provide any history due to altered mental status.

She is immediately brought to the ED resuscitation room, where she appears lethargic, unable to follow commands, diaphoretic, and with a subtle left-sided facial droop. Bradycardia, a cardiac murmur, and asymmetric pulses are noted in her lower extremities.

VITAL SIGNS

BP	110/40 mmHg
P	50 bpm
RR	18 breaths/min
O2	100% on 2L nasal cannula
T	36.9°C

DIFFERENTIAL DIAGNOSIS

Acute coronary syndrome
Aortic dissection
Arrhythmia
Cerebrovascular accident
Penetrating ulcer
Pericardial tamponade
Pneumothorax
Pulmonary embolism

POINT-OF-CARE ULTRASOUND was performed which showed the following:

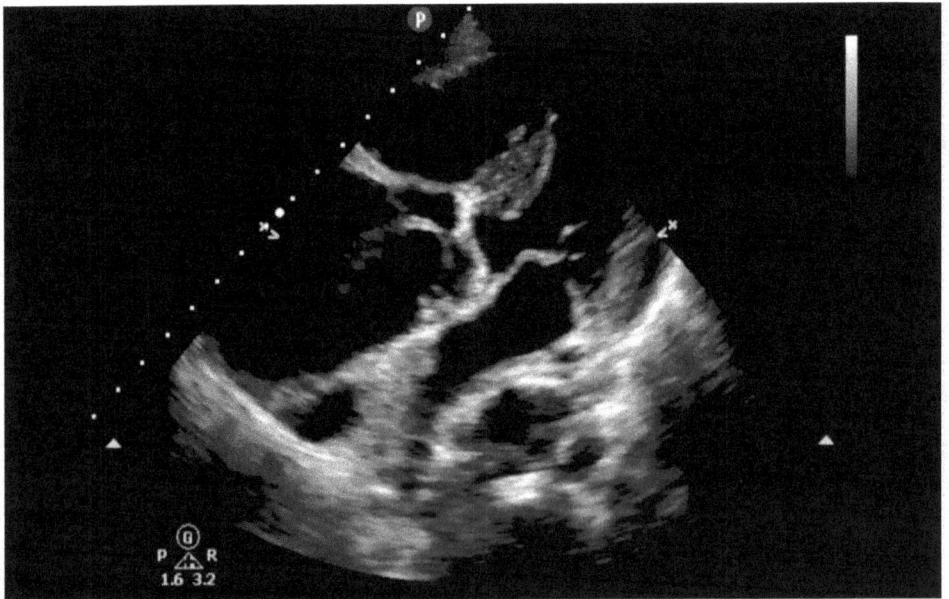

Figure 3.1

Parasternal long view of the heart revealing a thoracic aortic dissection

Figure 3.2

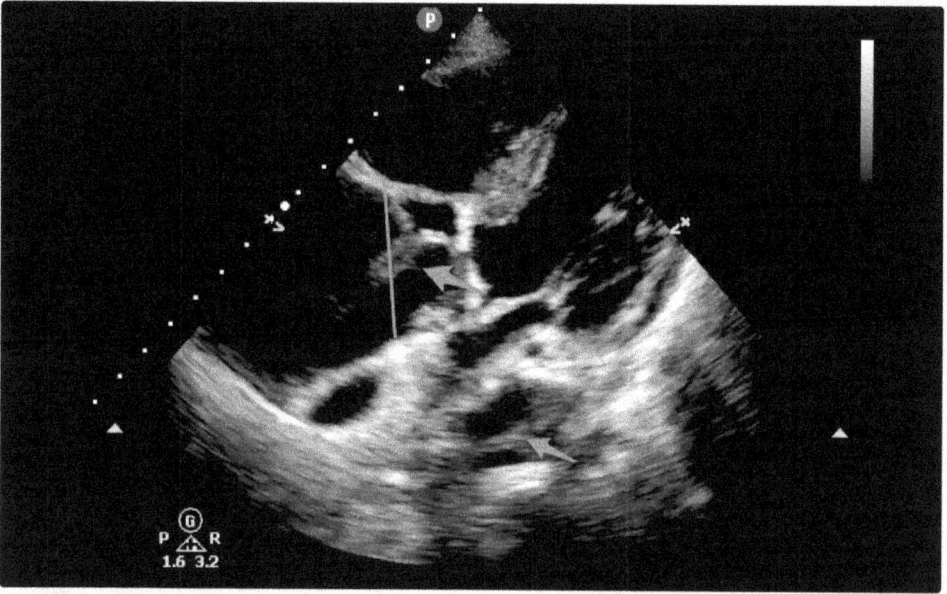

The bedside echocardiogram reveals a dilated aortic root (line) and visible dissection flaps (arrows).

The echocardiography findings (Fig. 3.1, 3.2.), in combination with the clinical scenario, is concerning for acute thoracic aortic dissection stemming from aneurysmal aortic disease.

ULTRASOUND IMAGE QUALITY ASSURANCE

An important aspect of ultrasound is appropriate and optimal image acquisition. The clip obtained is an adequate parasternal long axis (PLAX) view of the heart. This is obtained with the phased array probe placed at the 3rd-5th intercostal space just to the left of the sternum at the sterno-costal angle. The probe marker is oriented to the patient's right shoulder, at around 10 o'clock, which is typical of an ED echocardiogram (Fig 3.3). It is important to note that cardiology echocardiograms are done in an opposite probe indicator-to-screen orientation. For further discussion on this, please refer to Case 2, and the 2008 Moore paper [1], which is a must-read for anyone who performs echocardiograms.

Figure 3.3

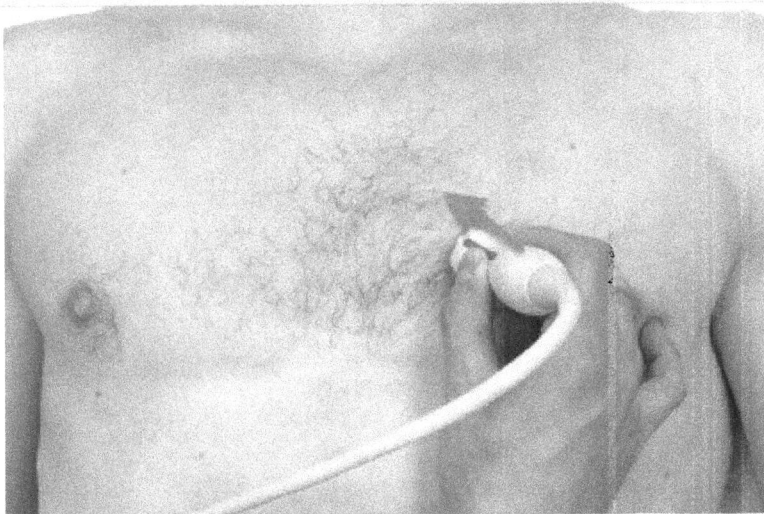

ED echocardiogram probe orientation. For the parasternal long axis (PLAX) view, the probe marker is oriented to the patient's right shoulder (arrow).

Figure 3.4

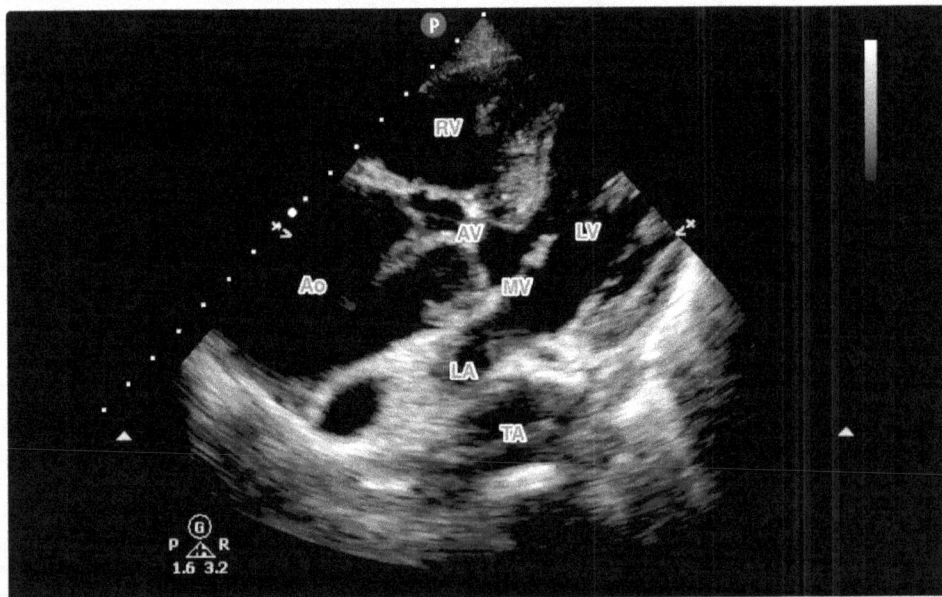

Labelled Parasternal Long Axis view of the heart

Several anatomic areas can be visualized in an ideal PLAX view (Figure 3.4): the left atrium (LA), mitral valves (MV), left ventricle (LV), aortic valves (AV), aortic root (Ao), right ventricle (RV), and descending thoracic aorta (TA).

In order to optimize the image, the depth should be increased slightly in order to completely visualize the cross-section of the descending thoracic aorta, allowing for measurement of the aortic diameter.

Lastly, thoracic aortic dissection is noted by the presence of the intimal flap, seen on the images at both the aortic root and descending thoracic aorta. Thoracic aortic dissection, while a distinct entity in itself, is often preceded by the presence of a thoracic aortic aneurysm. Thoracic aortic aneurysm is defined as a diameter > 4.0-4.5 cm, and is best identified in the parasternal long axis view. Measurements should be made at the largest visualized portion, from "leading edge to leading edge" [2]. To accomplish this, the calipers should be placed perpendicular to the axis of the vessel on the outside border of the aorta in the anterior field to the intimal surface of the posterior wall of the aorta in end-diastole.

Pearl: A suprasternal notch view can also visualize the aortic arch; however, this is out of the scope of this case series. More advanced techniques, such as color Doppler and spectral Doppler, can give further information about the flow (direction and velocity) in the true and false lumen.

DISPOSITION AND CASE CONCLUSION

The concerning findings on the bedside echocardiogram prompted the team to obtain a CT angiogram of the chest and abdomen which confirmed the diagnosis of an acute thoracic aortic dissection, with extensive aneurysmal dilatation of the ascending and descending thoracic aorta through to the abdominal aorta to below the level of the aortic bifurcation!

Given the high mortality associated with acute aortic dissection, the patient unfortunately did not survive her condition, but the expeditious workup allowed for the appropriate patient-centered management and goals of care discussions of this grave condition to occur in a timely manner.

Thoracic aortic aneurysms are less prevalent than abdominal aortic aneurysms, however the emergency physician must be able to be able to identify symptomatic thoracic aortic aneurysms [2]. Thoracic aneurysms are associated with aortic dissection, which if they occur have a high (>50%) mortality within the first 48 hours. Thus the diagnosis must be recognized quickly [3]. Bedside trans-thoracic echocardiogram is often the initial study of choice in many EDs for the evaluation of a patient with concern for aortic aneurysm or dissection given its ready availability, low cost, and lack of ionizing radiation. It is within the scope of the emergency physician to identify thoracic aortic pathology, as supported by consensus statements by the American College of Emergency Physicians and the American Society of Echocardiography [4].

It is important to recognize that the entire extent of the thoracic aorta cannot be entirely visualized with ultrasound, so if there is suspicion for a symptomatic aneurysm or dissection, a CT angiogram should be obtained. That being said, point-of-care echo can be a beneficial initial screening study. A recent retrospective study by Taylor et al. showed that a bedside trans-thoracic echocardiogram demonstrated good agreement with CT angiogram's measurements of maximal thoracic aortic diameter [5]. Thus, it is important to be aware of the echocardiographic findings that are suggestive of a thoracic aortic aneurysm (visualizing and measuring the aortic root, and descending thoracic aorta), and findings of a dissection (visible dissection flap).

TAKE-HOME POINTS

1. It is important to visualize regions of the thoracic aorta when performing a bedside trans-thoracic echocardiogram (TTE) to look for thoracic aneurysms or dissection.

2. Although important to obtain multiple views when performing a bedside echocardiogram, the parasternal long axis view is most ideal for visualization and measurement of portions of the thoracic aorta. Make sure you have enough depth to visualize the descending thoracic aorta.

3. Remember: The normal aortic root diameter is <4.0 cm. Larger than this suggests a thoracic aortic aneurysm and a possible ascending aortic dissection.

REFERENCES

1. Moore C. Current issues with emergency cardiac ultrasound probe and image conventions. Acad Emerg Med. 2008 Mar;15(3):278-84. PMID: 18304059.

2. Daignault MC, Saul T, Lewiss RE. Focused cardiac ultrasound diagnosis of thoracic aortic aneurysm: two cases. J Emerg Med. 2014 Mar;46(3):373-7. PMID: 23937808.

3. Mészáros I, Mórocz J, Szlávi J, Schmidt J, Tornóci L, Nagy L, Szép L. Epidemiology and clinicopathology of aortic dissection. Chest. 2000 May; 117(5):1271-8. PMID: 10807810.

4. Labovitz AJ, Noble VE, Bierig M, Goldstein SA, Jones R, Kort S, Porter TR, Spencer KT, Tayal VS, Wei K. Focused cardiac ultrasound in the emergent setting: a consensus statement of the American Society of Echocardiography and American College of Emergency Physicians. J Am Soc Echocardiogr. 2010 Dec;23(12):1225-30. PMID: 21111923.

5. Taylor RA, Oliva I, Van Tonder R, Elefteriades J, Dziura J, Moore CL. Point-of-care focused cardiac ultrasound for the assessment of thoracic aortic dimensions, dilation, and aneurysmal disease. Acad Emerg Med. 2012 Feb; 19(2): 244-7. PMID: 22288871.

22M with Scrotal Pain

OBJECTIVES

1. Identify the diagnostic utility of point-of-care ultrasonography in the patient presenting with acute scrotal pain.
2. Describe the ideal approach and patient positioning when performing a testicular point-of-care ultrasound.
3. Describe the findings of testicular torsion seen with point-of-care ultrasound.
4. Define Resistive Index (RI), the normal range of values, and the significance to a testicular ultrasound.

CASE PRESENTATION

A 22-year-old otherwise healthy man presents to the ED with an acute onset of right testicular pain. He states his pain started about 2.5 hours prior to arrival in the ED. He has associated nausea, but no vomiting. He denies any recent sexual activity or trauma. The remainder of the history is unremarkable. On exam, he appears to be in moderate distress, and he has exquisite tenderness to palpation and moderate swelling of the right testicle. The left testicle is non-tender and unremarkable.

VITAL SIGNS

BP	119/82 mmHg
P	109 bpm
RR	22 breaths/min
O2	99% room air
T	37.2°C

DIFFERENTIAL DIAGNOSIS

Epididymitis
Hematoma
Hernia
Hydrocele
Orchitis
Mass / Tumor
Testicular torsion
Scrotal abscess
Varicocele

POINT-OF-CARE ULTRASOUND was performed which showed the following:

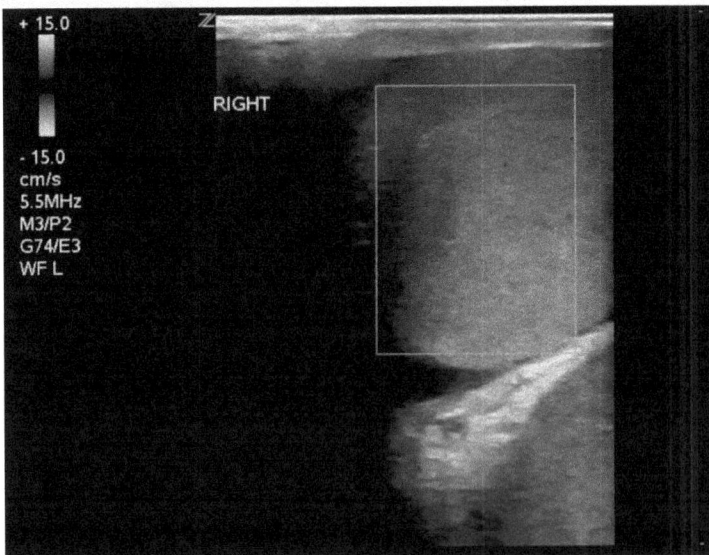

Figure 4.1

Ultrasound of the right testicle showing no flow is seen with color Doppler.

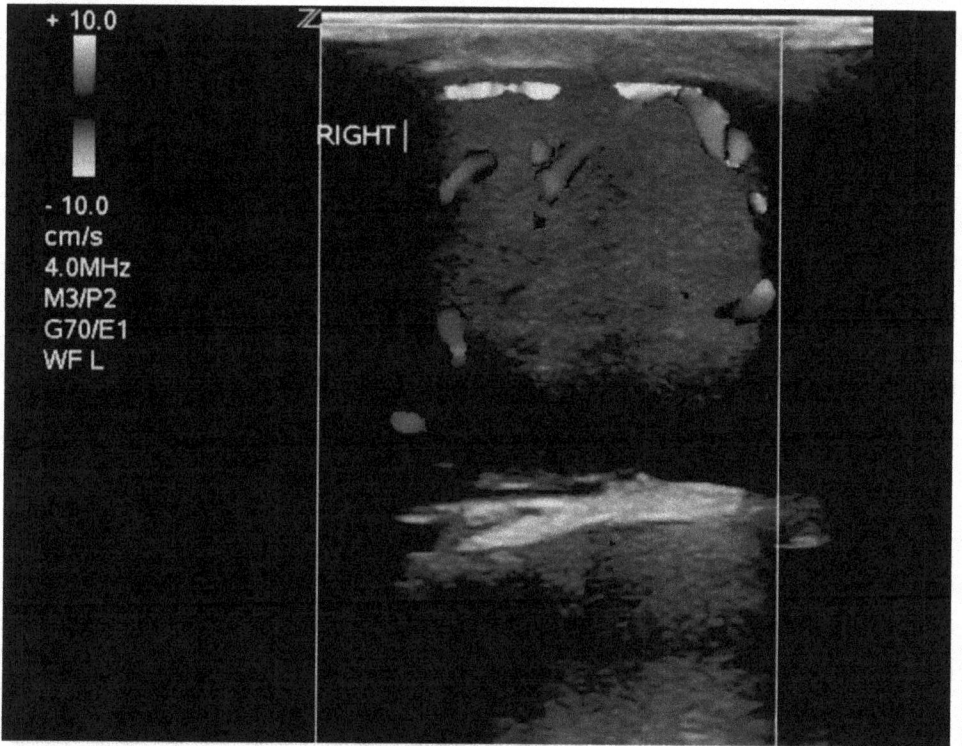

Figure 4.2

Repeat ultrasound of the right testicle after manual detorsion showing reperfusion hyperemia as visualized with color Doppler

The right testicle in Fig. 4.1 is concerning for testicular torsion with there being a lack of blood flow to the testicle on color Doppler. Given the emergent nature of the condition, urology was consulted, and the testicle was manually detorsed by the emergency physician using the "open book" technique with relief of symptoms. Immediate repeat point-of-care ultrasound of the right testicle with color Doppler (Fig. 4.2) revealed reperfusion hyperemia. This is commonly seen after a testicle is detorsed.

ULTRASOUND IMAGE QUALITY ASSURANCE

The ultrasound images in this case were obtained using a high-frequency linear probe. A general approach is to have the patient comfortably sitting or laying supine in a frog-leg position. A rolled towel can be draped under the scrotum to elevate and stabilize the testicles. Warm gel should ideally be used for comfort. A tegaderm can be placed over the linear probe to keep the probe clean.

Once the patient is positioned, it is best to start with the non-affected testicle for patient comfort as well as providing a baseline for the ultrasonographer. The gain, depth, and color Doppler scale can be adjusted until just enough color Doppler flow is obtained with minimal background noise.

Tip: Using your ultrasound machine's "auto calibrate" button will usually suffice to optimize this for you!.

The use of color Doppler to visualize testicular blood flow has been shown to be highly sensitive (86%) and specific (100%) in aiding in the diagnosis of testicular torsion when assessing for the presence or absence of intratesticular blood flow [1].

If you reach the lowest scale using color Doppler and are still unable to visualize testicular blood flow, switching to power Doppler may help. Power Doppler is up to five times more sensitive for low-flow states than color Doppler [2], and is less dependent on angle. A testicle with normal color Doppler flow is shown (Fig. 4.3):

Figure 4.3

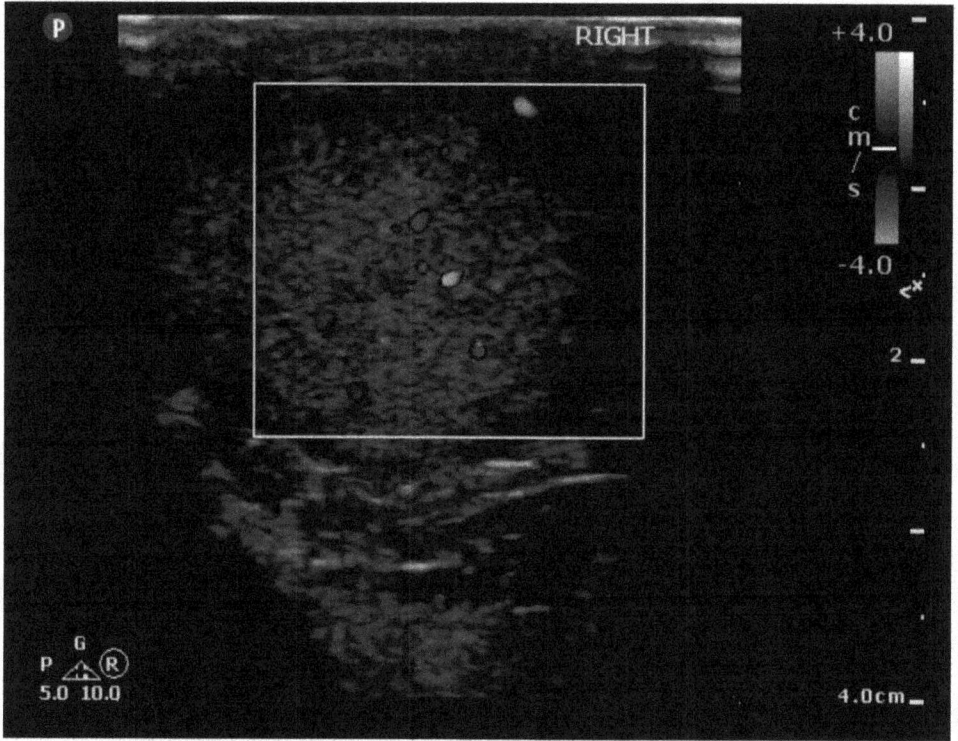

Normal testicular ultrasound showing the normal homogenous echotexture and normal flow pattern with color Doppler.

For advanced readers:

In addition to simply looking qualitatively at the blood flow with color Doppler, a Resistive Index (RI) can be measured. Using pulsed-wave spectral Doppler with the gate positioned over a testicular artery, an arterial waveform is produced. The Resistive Index can then be calculated using the formula:

$$RI = \frac{\text{(Peak Systolic Velocity–End Diastolic Velocity)}}{\text{Peak Systolic Velocity}}$$

Most ultrasound machines will be able to calculate this for you. A normal testicular RI is 0.5-0.7 [3]; an RI higher than this suggests an increased resistance to flow which can be concerning for early torsion.

Pulsed-wave Doppler (Fig. 4.4) with the gate (=) positioned over a testicular vessel produces a waveform from which the peak systolic velocity (SV) and end diastolic velocity (DV) can be measured. In this particular image, the RI is 0.635 cm/s, which is normal.

As with most point-of-care ultrasound, scan the testicle in two planes, including the epididymis, and assess the echotexture. Once a baseline is obtained from the unaffected testicle, you can move on to the affected testicle in the same manner, using the settings you have just optimized. For testicular torsion, you are looking

---

Figure 4.4

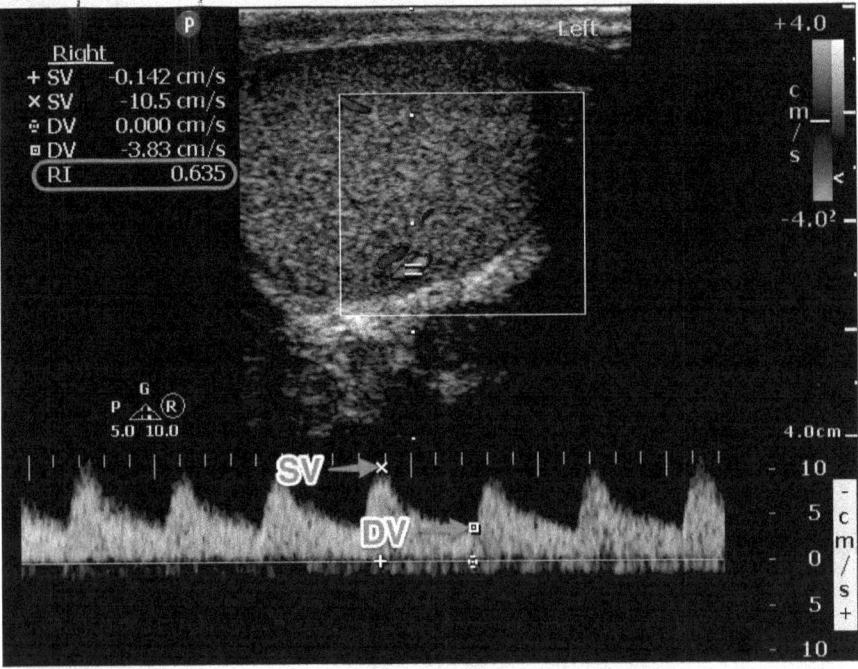

Measurement of Resistive Index of a testicular vessel using pulsed-wave spectral Doppler

specifically for lack of blood flow, or a high resistive index.

DISPOSITION AND CASE CONCLUSION

Given the findings of testicular torsion confirmed with bedside ultrasound, urology was emergently consulted, and the patient was taken to the operating room for orchiopexy. The testicle was salvaged. The patient has since been discharged and is doing well.

Testicular torsion has an incidence of 1 in 4,000 males, with pubescent boys being most frequently affected [4]. Torsion is a cause of significant morbidity with average testicular salvage rates being low at only 50% [4]. It is often said that "time is testicle", with signs of testicular hemorrhage and infarction appearing within 2 hours of testicular artery occlusion, and irreversible ischemia after 6 hours [5]. Thus, it is important to diagnose testicular torsion as early as possible to reduce time to definitive surgical management, and have urology consulted as soon as torsion is considered.

Color Doppler ultrasonography is considered the imaging mode of choice in patients presenting with acute scrotal pain. Given the time-sensitive nature of testicular emergencies such as testicular torsion, it is extremely valuable for an emergency physician to have the skill to perform point-of-care testicular ultrasonography. This is especially beneficial in smaller community EDs where prompt radiology-performed ultrasonography may not be readily available. An point-of-care ultrasound can be performed easily and promptly in patients who present to the ED with acute scrotal pain with high sensitivity (95%) and specificity (94%) [6]. As seen in this case, it can aid in the diagnosis of testicular torsion, and can expedite time to definitive surgical management.

TAKE-HOME POINTS

1. Testicular ultrasound can aid in the diagnosis of acute scrotal pathology, and is a useful skill for emergency physicians.

2. Point-of-care testicular ultrasonography by emergency physicians has a high sensitivity (95%) and specificity (94%) [6].

3. Start with the unaffected testicle to optimize your settings. The auto-calibrate button can help!

4. Resistive Index = (Peak Systolic Velocity-End Diastolic Velocity)/Peak Systolic Velocity. The normal range is 0.5-0.7 cm/sec.

5. Testicular torsion is a surgical emergency. Call the urologist as soon as it is suspected.

REFERENCES

1. Burks DD, Markey BJ, Burkhard TK, Balsara ZN, Haluszka MM, Canning DA. Suspected testicular torsion and ischemia: evaluation with color Doppler sonography. Radiology. 1990 Jun;175(3):815-21. PMID: 2188301.

2. Blaivas M, Brannam L. Testicular ultrasound. Emerg Med Clin North Am. 2004 Aug;22(3):723-48, ix. PMID: 15301848.

3. Carmody et al. Handbook of Critical Care & Emergency Ultrasound. 2011.

4. Blaivas M, Batts M, Lambert M. Ultrasonographic diagnosis of testicular torsion by emergency physicians. Am J Emerg Med. 2000 Mar;18(2):198-200. PMID: 10750932.

5. Luker GD, Siegel MJ. Color Doppler sonography of the scrotum in children. Am J Roentgenol 1994; 163:649-655. PMID: 8079863.

6. Blaivas M, Sierzenski P, Lambert M. Emergency evaluation of patients presenting with acute scrotum using bedside ultrasonography. Acad Emerg Med. 2001 Jan;8(1):90-3. PMID: 11136159.

30M with Blunt Abdominal Trauma

OBJECTIVES

1. Define the FAST examination and its utility in the Emergency Department.
2. List the limitations of the FAST examination for certain types of traumatic injuries.
3. Describe the major findings of the SOAP trial and its significance to patients who present to the Emergency Department with trauma.

CASE PRESENTATION

A 30-year-old male is brought in by paramedics after a high-speed motor vehicle collision where an automobile crashed into a stationary pole. Two other passengers died in the field. Per report, the patient was approximately 15 feet (4.6 meters) from the vehicle, which suffered major damage.

The patient is immediately brought into the trauma bay, where he is confused but follows commands. He has an obvious humerus fracture. His Glasgow Coma Scale score is 14, and he is moving all extremities. Other than his depressed mental status, the primary survey is unrevealing.

VITAL SIGNS

BP	133/88 mmHg
P	132 bpm
RR	28 breaths/min
O2	100% on 2L nasal cannula
T	37.1°C

DIFFERENTIAL DIAGNOSIS

Cervical spine or other spinal injury
Hollow viscous (bowel) injury
Intracranial injury
Pelvic or other orthopedic injuries
Pneumothorax
Solid organ injury
Thoracic injury

POINT-OF-CARE ULTRASOUND was performed which showed the following:

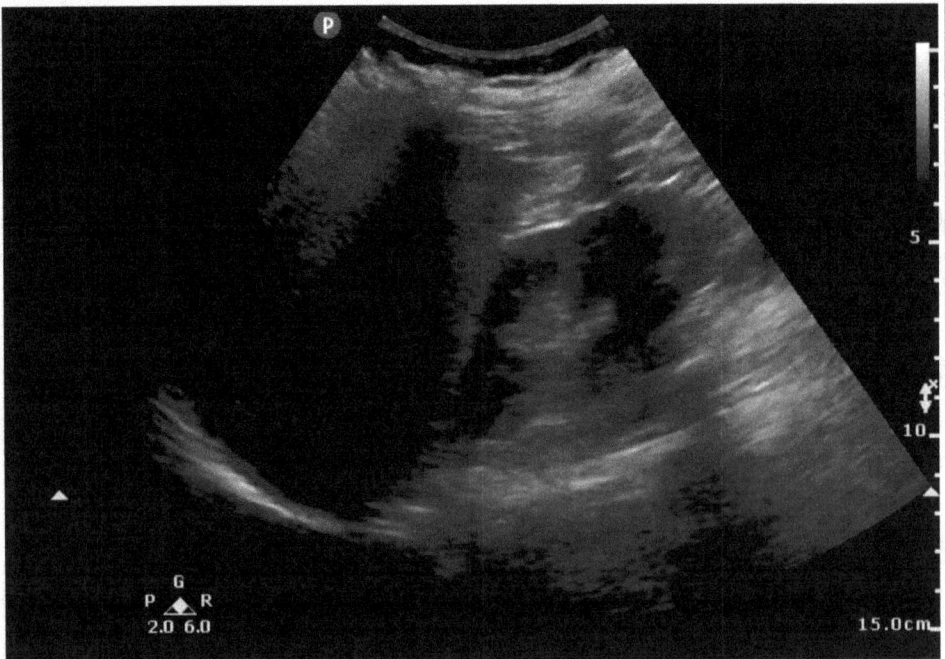

Figure 5.1

Right upper quadrant view of the FAST exam

Figure 5.2

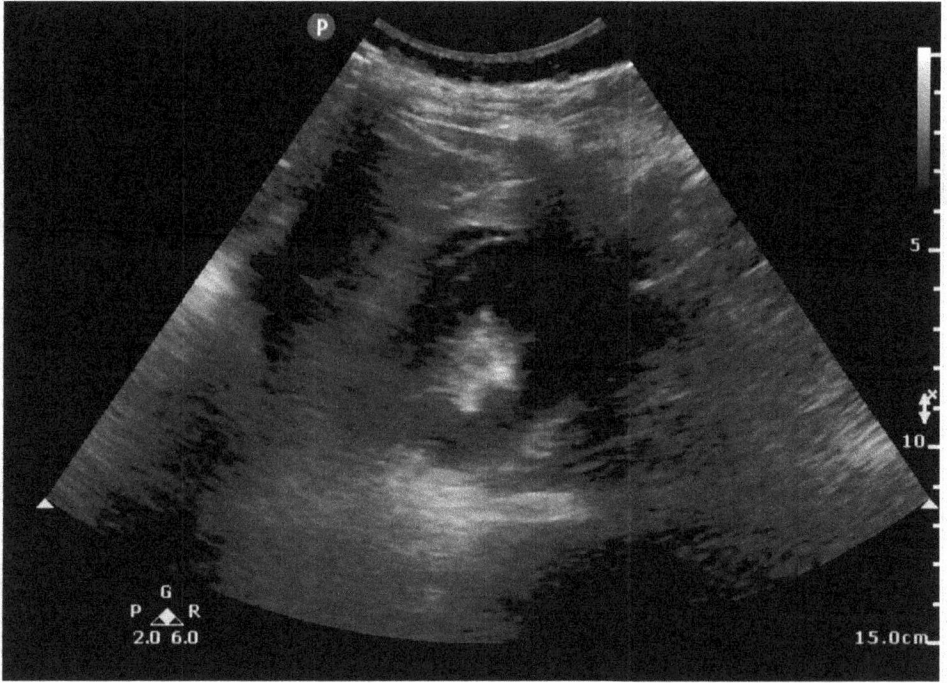

Left upper quadrant view of the FAST exam

A Focused Assessment with Sonography in Trauma (FAST) was performed. The right upper quadrant (RUQ) view (Fig. 5.1) appears negative for free fluid, but there is a small fluid collection seen in the left upper quadrant (LUQ) (Fig. 5.2, 5.3).

ULTRASOUND IMAGE QUALITY ASSURANCE

An important aspect of ultrasound is appropriate and optimal image acquisition. The clips, showing only the RUQ and LUQ portions of the FAST, demonstrate appropriate gain and probe orientation. The depth in the clip of the RUQ is

Figure 5.3

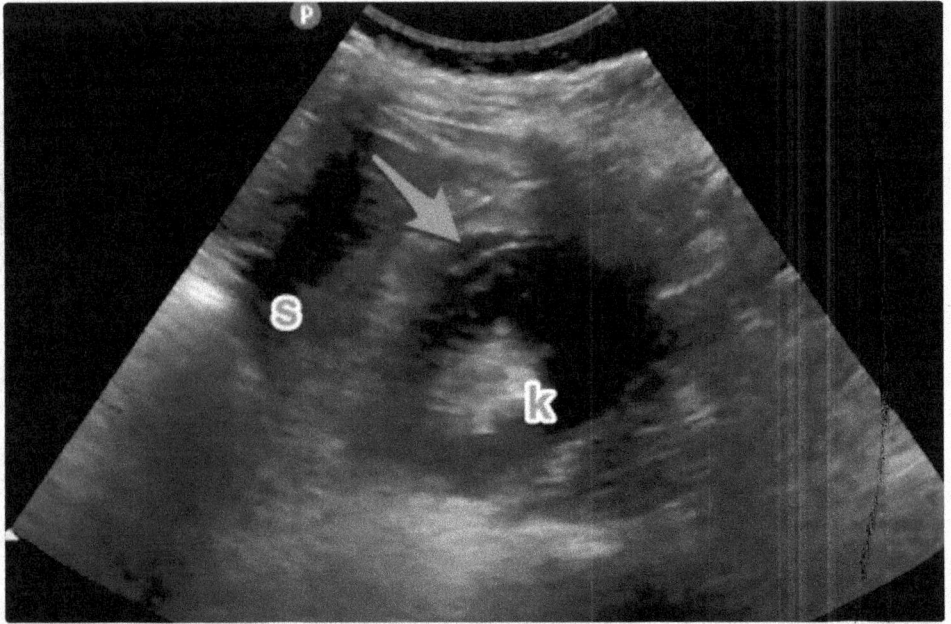

Left upper quadrant view of the FAST exam with labels showing the presence of free fluid (arrow).
(s=spleen, k=kidney)

optimal, with visualization of not only Morison's pouch, but also of the paracolic gutter, and above the diaphragm looking for potential hemothorax. Unfortunately, the left hemidiaphragm on the LUQ view is not well visualized in the clip. Additionally, the depth on the LUQ view could be decreased somewhat in order to maximize the use of the focal zone and improve the image quality.

The curvilinear (aka "abdominal") probe was used for the FAST exam. Given its relatively large footprint, several rib shadows were visualized in the clips. While insignificant in this case, sometimes rib shadows can obscure areas of interest. There are two tips to help avoid rib shadows.

Tip #1: Rotate the probe slightly from the coronal plane to run more parallel to the ribs, positioning the ultrasound beam between the ribs.

Tip #2: Use the phased array (aka "cardiac") probe, which has a smaller footprint to maneuver between the rib spaces.

A common pitfall of the RUQ view is visualizing only the interface between the liver and kidney (Morison's pouch); however, it is important to assess the caudal tip of the liver, which is more sensitive for smaller fluid collections as they tend to begin there before tracking into Morison's pouch [1]. Additionally, in the LUQ view, it is important to not only visualize the splenorenal interface, but also the interface between the diaphragm and the spleen.

DISPOSITION AND CASE CONCLUSION

Shortly after the FAST was performed, the patient became hypotensive. Fortunately, he responded to fluids. Since he was hemodynamically stable, the decision was made to proceed to the CT scanner. CT imaging revealed a shattered spleen with multiple lacerations. Hemoperitoneum was noted around the spleen, extending to the right paracolic gutter and perihepatic region.

The patient was taken to the operating room by the trauma surgery team. Intra-operatively, he was noted to have a fractured spleen, as well as a large retroperitoneal hematoma. A splenectomy was performed, and serosal tears were repaired. The patient remained hemodynamically stable in the surgical intensive care uni, and was eventually discharged from the hospital. He is currently at home, and is doing well!

A FAST examination is a quick and non-invasive study that can easily be performed in patients who present with blunt or penetrating trauma. It is sensitive and specific for the identification of hemoperitoneum in the abdomen and pelvis as well as for pericardial effusion. A meta-analysis of 62 trials, which included more than 18,000 patients, showed a pooled sensitivity of 78.9% and specificity of 99.2% [2].

The SOAP trial, a multicenter randomized controlled trial by Melniker et al. showed that the FAST exam decreases time to operative care, reduces the number of CT scans ordered, decreases patient morbidity, and shortens hospital length of stay [3]. This case demonstrates the high utility of a bedside FAST exam for trauma patients who present to the ED.

An E-FAST (Extended FAST) includes thoracic views for identifying potential pneumothorax or hemothorax, and has been shown to be more accurate than x-ray in identifying these pathologies [4,5].

Limitations of the FAST Exam

While the FAST is a useful tool in the evaluation of the trauma patient, physicians must be aware of its strengths as well as its limitations. These limitations include the inability to detect certain types of injuries, such as injury to the bowel or diaphragm, retroperitoneal hemorrhage, and vascular injuries [6]. Furthermore, a FAST relies on hemoperitoneum, so solid organ injury without evidence of hemoperitoneum will potentially be missed [7]. Thus, if there is a high clinical suspicion of intra-abdominal injuries despite a negative FAST, further studies such as serial FAST exams or CT should be considered in the hemodynamically stable patient.

TAKE-HOME POINTS

1. The FAST exam has a sensitivity of 78.9% and high specificity of 99.2%, highlighting that while smaller amounts of free fluid may be missed, if seen, it is highly accurate for an intra-abdominal injury in the setting of trauma [3].

2. Positive FAST + hemodynamic instability = Operating Room!

3. A point-of-care FAST exam in the ED in the trauma patient decreases time to definitive operative care, improved resource use (fewer CT studies), and reduces patient morbidity [2].

4. Limitations of the FAST exam include: limited detection for certain types of injuries (bowel, retroperitoneal, vascular), and abdominal injury without hemoperitoneum [6,7].

REFERENCES

1. Williams SR, Perera P, Gharahbaghian L. The FAST and E-FAST in 2013: trauma ultrasonography: overview, practical techniques, controversies, and new frontiers. Crit Care Clin. 2014 Jan;30(1):119-50, vi. PMID: 24295843.

2. Stengel D, Bauwens K, Rademacher G, Mutze S, Ekkernkamp A. Association between compliance with methodological standards of diagnostic research and reported test accuracy: meta-analysis of focused assessment of US for trauma. Radiology. 2005 Jul;236(1):102-11. PMID: 15983072.

3. Melniker LA, Leibner E, McKenney MG, Lopez P, Briggs WM, Mancuso CA. Randomized controlled clinical trial of point-of-care, limited ultrasonography for trauma in the emergency department: the first sonography outcomes assessment program trial. Ann Emerg Med. 2006 Sep;48(3):227-35. PMID: 16934640.

4. Brooks A, Davies B, Smethhurst M, Connolly J. Emergency ultrasound in the acute assessment of haemothorax. Emerg Med J. 2004 Jan;21(1):44-6. PMID: 14734374.

5. Blaivas M, Lyon M, Duggal S. A prospective comparison of supine chest radiography and bedside ultrasound for the diagnosis of traumatic pneumothorax. Acad Emerg Med. 2005 Sep;12(9):844-9. PMID: 16141018.

6. Tsui CL, Fung HT, Chung KL, Kam CW. Focused abdominal sonography for trauma in the emergency department for blunt abdominal trauma. Int J Emerg Med. 2008 Sep;1(3):183-7. PMID: 19384513.

7. Chiu WC, Cushing BM, Rodriguez A, Ho SM, Mirvis SE, Shanmuganathan K, Stein M. Abdominal injuries without hemoperitoneum: a potential limitation of focused abdominal sonography for trauma (FAST). J Trauma. 1997 Apr; 42(4):617-23; discussion 623-5. PMID: 9137247.

46F with Abdominal Pain

OBJECTIVES

1. Summarize the test characteristics of CT imaging compared to ultrasound in assessing gallbladder pathology.
2. Describe the sonographic appearance of stones on ultrasound.
3. Identify the normal sonographic landmarks when attempting to visualize the gallbladder.
4. List the four sonographic findings of cholecystitis.
5. Define the "Stone-in-Neck" ultrasound sign and its significance.

CASE PRESENTATION

A 46-year-old obese woman presents to the ED with 3 hours of non-bilious emesis and right-sided abdominal pain. She has been unable to eat secondary to pain. On examination, she appears to be in moderate distress, and has diffuse abdominal tenderness to palpation, worst at the right upper quadrant without rebound or guarding.

VITAL SIGNS

BP	127/77 mmHg
P	112 bpm
RR	20 breaths/min
O2	99% room air
T	36.6°C

DIFFERENTIAL DIAGNOSIS

Appendicitis
Cholangitis
Cholecystitis
Choledocolithiasis
Cholelithiasis
Gastritis
Pancreatic mass
Pancreatitis
Peptic ulcer disease
Pregnancy
Viral syndrome

INITIAL WORKUP

A computed tomography (CT) of the abdomen and pelvis with intravenous contrast was obtained. The radiology report was read as normal.

Labs:
- White blood cells: 10.4 cells/hpf
- Total bilirubin: 1.6 mg/dL
- Direct bilirubin: 1.2 mg/dL
- Alkaline phosphatase: 274 U/L
- Alanine aminotransferase (ALT): 464 IU/L
- Aspartate aminotransferase (AST): 447 IU/L
- Urinalysis: Negative for pregnancy, leukocytes, nitrites, white blood cells, and red blood cells

Given the ongoing concern for potential gallbladder pathology, a point-of-care ultrasound was performed.

POINT-OF-CARE ULTRASOUND was performed which showed the following:

Figure 6.1

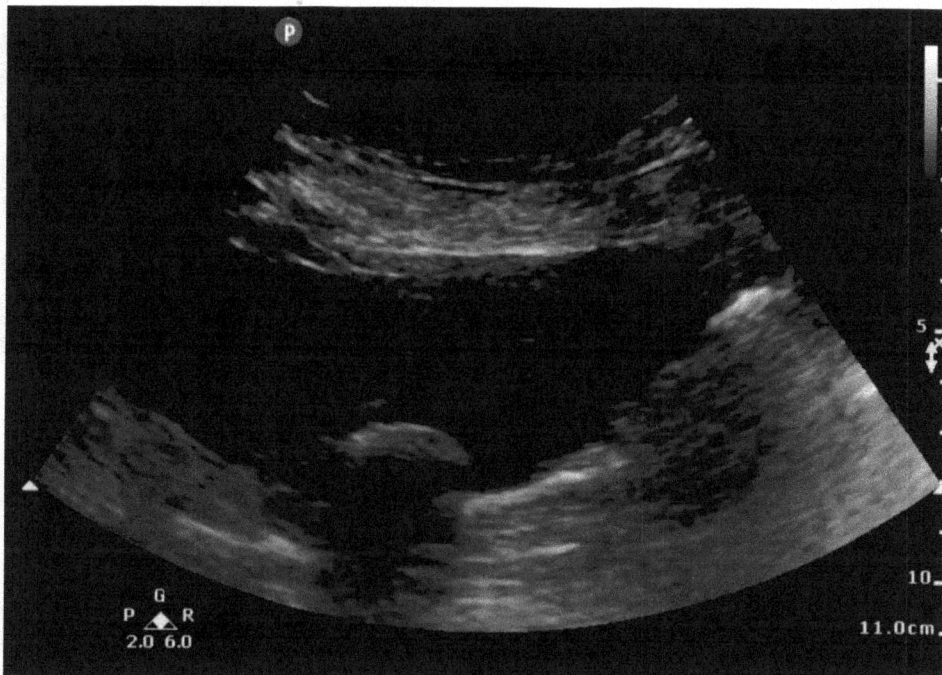

Point-of-care ultrasound of the gallbladder showing a large stone in the gallbladder neck (Stone-in-Neck sign), concerning for acute cholecystitis

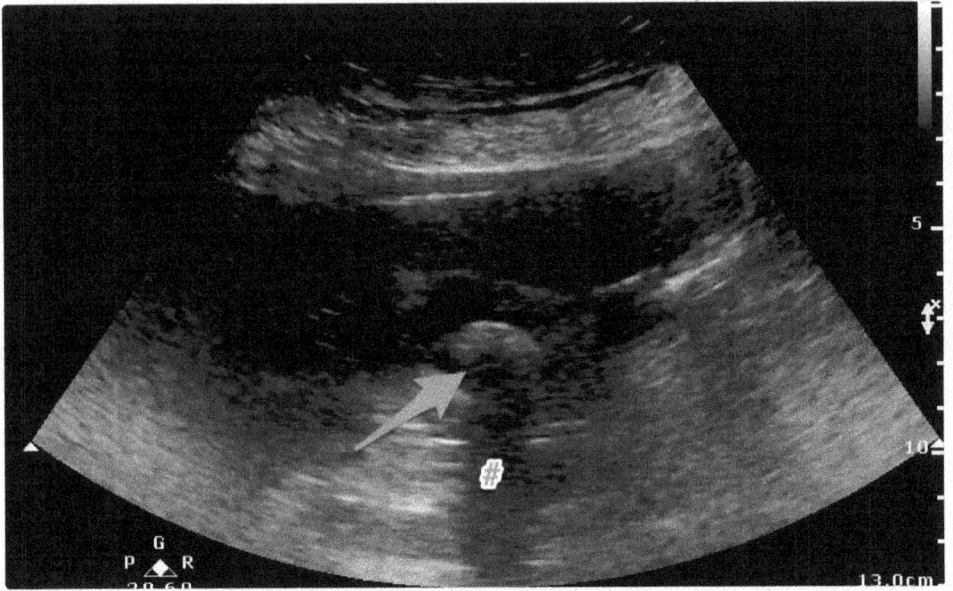

Figure 6.2

The Stone-in-Neck sign: An immobile hyperechoic stone (arrow) seen in the gallbladder neck with posterior shadowing (#)

The images in this case (Fig. 6.1, 6.2) demonstrate a stone lodged in the neck of the gallbladder – also known as the "Stone-in-Neck" (SIN) sign [1]. A large hyperechoic stone is seen with posterior shadowing. Rolling the patient to left and right lateral positions may be necessary to distinguish between a mobile versus a non-mobile stone in the neck. A SIN sign is highly suggestive of cholecystitis, and has been found to be 97% specific [1].

ULTRASOUND IMAGE QUALITY ASSURANCE

Point-of-care ultrasonography of the gallbladder is one of the more challenging bedside studies to perform. This study is ideally performed with the curvilinear probe; the lower frequency of this probe allows for greater penetration that can be helpful, especially in obese patients.

There are a few ways to identify the gallbladder.

- Start in a sagittal plane at the subxiphoid and slide the probe inferiorly and to the patient's right just below the costal margin, or

- Start at the mid-axillary line on the patient's right side in a coronal orientation, similar to a FAST study.

- Having the patient take a breath in and holding it, or turning them onto their left lateral side may also optimize positioning to help to visualize the gallbladder.

Once visualized, the gallbladder anatomy should be identified including the fundus, body, and neck (Fig. 6.3). As is the case with most point-of-care ultrasound studies, you should obtain images in two planes to avoid missing potential pathology. The main lobar fissure (MLF), seen as a bright hyperechoic line, is a landmark that allows for identification of the portal triad, and together has the appearance of an exclamation point.

The next step is to visualize potential gallbladder pathology including cholelithiasis or acute cholecystitis (Fig. 6.4).

Figure 6.3

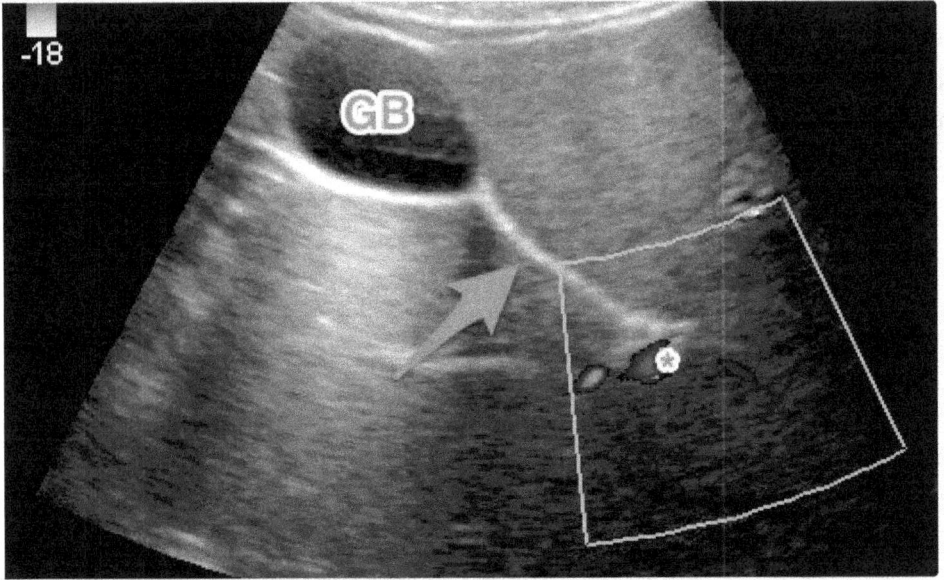

Landmarks for the gallbladder (GB) include the main lobar fissure (arrow) which extends from the GB to the portal triad (*)

Figure 6.4

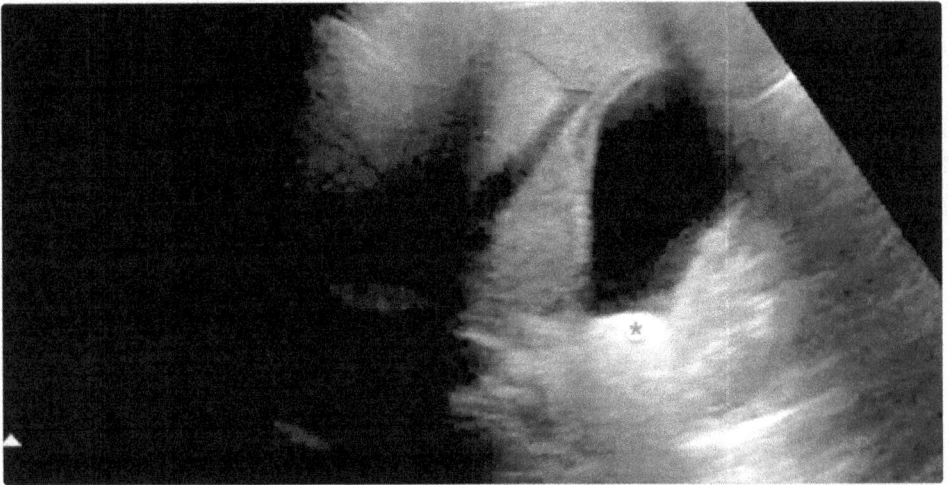

Sonographic signs of acute cholecystitis includes visualizing a gallbladder with a hyperechoic stone, wall thickening, and pericholecystic fluid (arrow)

The **4 SONOGRAPHIC SIGNS OF CHOLECYSTITIS** are:

1. **Gallstones/Sludge** – Visualized as hyperechoic structures within the gallbladder with posterior shadowing.
2. **Thickened Gallbladder Wall** – Wall thickness >4 mm. Of note, the anterior, not posterior wall, should be measured to avoid overestimating of the wall due to artifacts off the posterior wall.
3. **Pericholecystic Fluid** – Seen as an anechoic stripe surrounding the gallbladder.
4. **Sonographic Murphy Sign** – Reproduction of pain when pressure is applied directly over the visualized gallbladder using the ultrasound probe.

Although all four signs are not needed to make a diagnosis of cholecystitis, the presence of all four signs is very specific for cholecystitis. Conversely, each sign seen independently is non-specific and should be taken into context with the clinical scenario.

DISPOSITION AND CASE CONCLUSION

General surgery was consulted given the concerning findings on ultrasound, and the patient was admitted to the hospital for further management.

Point-of-care ultrasonography of the right upper quadrant is an important skill for the emergency physician to have. The initial CT scan was read as negative, and if the provider had been falsely reassured by that and discharged the patient, it would have likely led to a bad outcome.

This case highlights the fact that ultrasonography is superior to CT for the evaluation of gallbladder pathology. While the CT scan revealed no evidence of cholelithiasis or cholecystitis, the point-of-care ultrasound revealed a large stone in the neck ("Stone-in-Neck sign") which is highly suggestive for cholecystitis. Ultrasonography has been shown to be more sensitive for the identification of cholelithiasis and cholecystitis. CT imaging is 79.1% sensitive and 100% specific for cholelithiasis [2], compared with 88% sensitivity and 87% specificity with ED-performed point-of-care ultrasonography [3].

As radiology-performed ultrasound may be limited or unavailable at smaller community EDs, it is important for the EP to have the skills to identify acute cholecystitis on point-of-care ultrasound. EP-performed ultrasonography for the diagnosis of acute cholecystitis has been shown in a prospective study to be not significantly different from radiology-performed ultrasound (87% sensitive and 82% specific for ED ultrasound, compared with 83% sensitive and 86% specific for radiology ultrasound) using pathology specimens as the gold standard [4].

TAKE-HOME POINTS

1. Point-of-care ultrasonography of the right upper quadrant is an essential skill for the emergency physician. It is more sensitive than CT for evaluation of gallbladder pathology.

2. Sonographic findings of cholecystitis include:

   - Gallstones/sludge
   - Thickened gallbladder wall
   - Pericholecystic fluid
   - Sonographic Murphy Sign

3. The Stone-in-Neck sign, visualization of an immobile stone lodged in the neck of the gallbladder, is highly suggestive of acute cholecystitis with 97% specificity [1].

REFERENCES

1. Nelson M, Ash A, Raio C, Zimmerman M. Stone-In-Neck phenomenon: a new sign of cholecystitis. Crit Ultrasound J. 2011;3(2):115-117. doi: 10.1007/s13089-011-0071-6.

2. Barakos JA, Ralls PW, Lapin SA, Johnson MB, Radin DR, Colletti PM, Boswell WD Jr, Halls JM. Cholelithiasis: evaluation with CT. Radiology. 1987 Feb; 162(2):415-8. PMID: 3797654.

3. Scruggs W, Fox JC, Potts B, Zlidenny A, McDonough J, Anderson CL, Larson J, Barajas G, Langdorf MI. Accuracy of ED Bedside Ultrasound for Identification of gallstones: retrospective analysis of 575 studies. West J Emerg Med. 2008 Jan;9(1):1-5. PMID: 19561694.

4. Summers SM, Scruggs W, Menchine MD, Lahham S, Anderson C, Amr O, Lotfipour S, Cusick SS, Fox JC. A prospective evaluation of emergency department bedside ultrasonography for the detection of acute cholecystitis. Ann Emerg Med. 2010 Aug;56(2):114-22. PMID: 20138397.

39F with Chest Pain

OBJECTIVES

1. Describe the utility of point-of-care ultrasound in patients presenting with shock.
2. Identify the difference between a pericardial effusion versus a pleural effusion on ultrasound.
3. List two pitfalls that can be mistaken for a pericardial effusion on ultrasound.
4. Discuss the importance of obtaining multiple views of the heart when assessing for a pericardial effusion.
5. Describe the echocardiographic findings of pericardial tamponade.

CASE PRESENTATION

A 39-year-old female with systemic lupus erythematosus presents to the ED by ambulance for evaluation of chest pain. Of note, she was recently discharged from the hospital for pneumonia with an exudative pleural effusion. Per the paramedic report, she was noted to be hypotensive with systolic blood pressures in the 70s. Two peripheral IV's were started with IV fluids running. A prehospital electrocardiogram rhythm strip revealed a narrow complex tachycardia.

On examination, the patient is distressed, tachypneic, and has distended neck veins.

VITAL SIGNS

BP	90/60 mmHg
P	146 bpm
RR	31 breaths/min
O2	96% on 15L oxygen via non-rebreather face mask
T	36.8°C

DIFFERENTIAL DIAGNOSIS

Acute coronary syndrome
Arrhythmia
Pericardial tamponade
Pleural effusion
Pneumonia
Pneumothorax
Pulmonary embolism

A patient who presents to the ED with chest pain in shock has a broad differential diagnosis list, several of which are noted above. The rapid use of one of many bedside ultrasound-guided protocols, such as Rapid Ultrasound for Shock and Hypotension (RUSH) [1] or Abdominal and Cardiac Evaluation with Sonography in Shock (ACES) [2], can be used to aid in narrowing your differential and finding potential reversible causes of shock. These protocols usually combine a few focused exams, including echocardiogram, inferior vena cava (IVC), thoracic, and aorta. In this case, an echocardiogram was performed first.

POINT-OF-CARE ULTRASOUND was performed which showed the following:

Figure 7.1

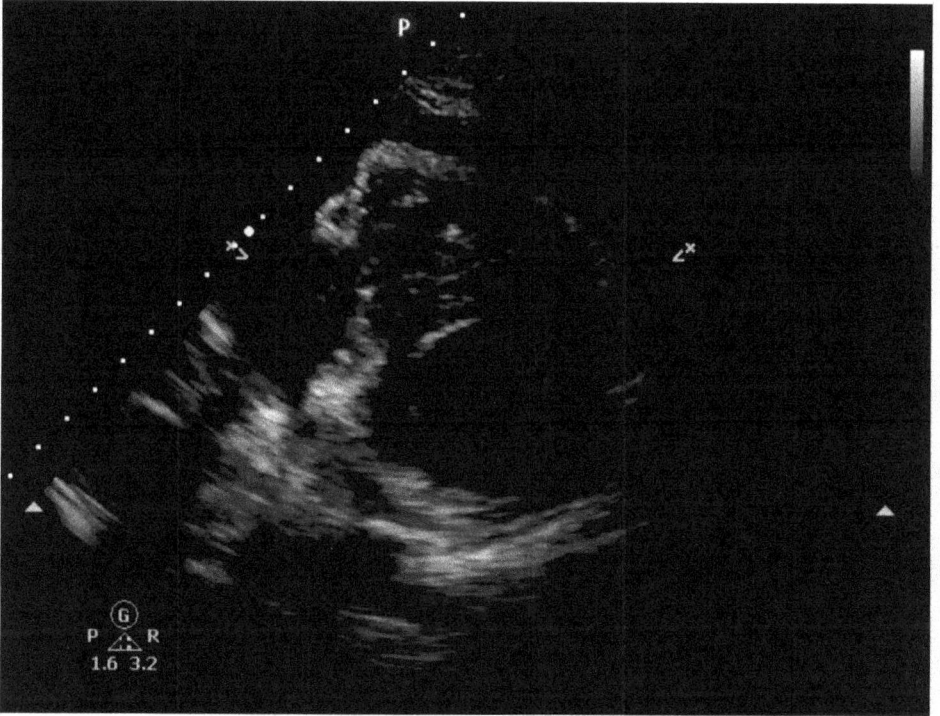

Parasternal short axis of the heart revealing a large pericardial effusion with echocardiographic signs of cardiac tamponade

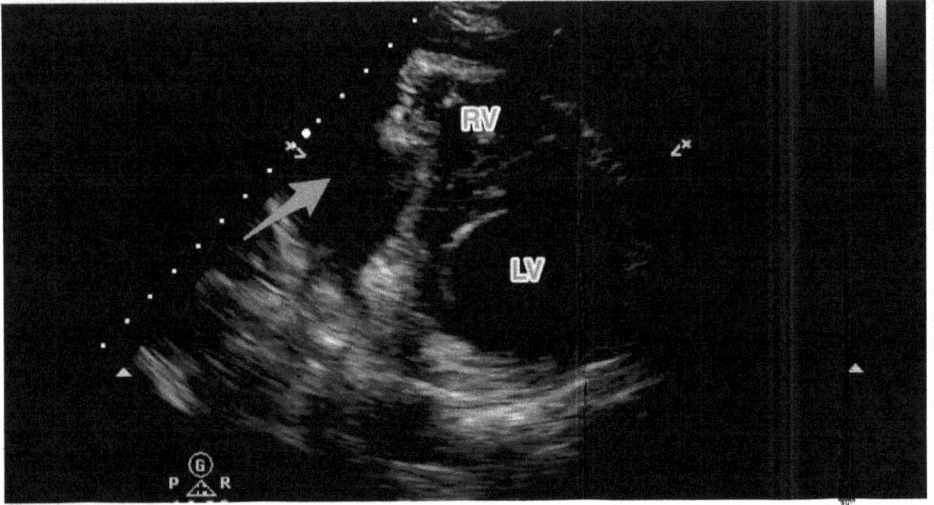

Figure 7.2

Labelled image from Figure 7.1 showing the large pericardial effusion (arrow) with right ventricular (RV) collapse. Also seen is the left ventricle (LV).

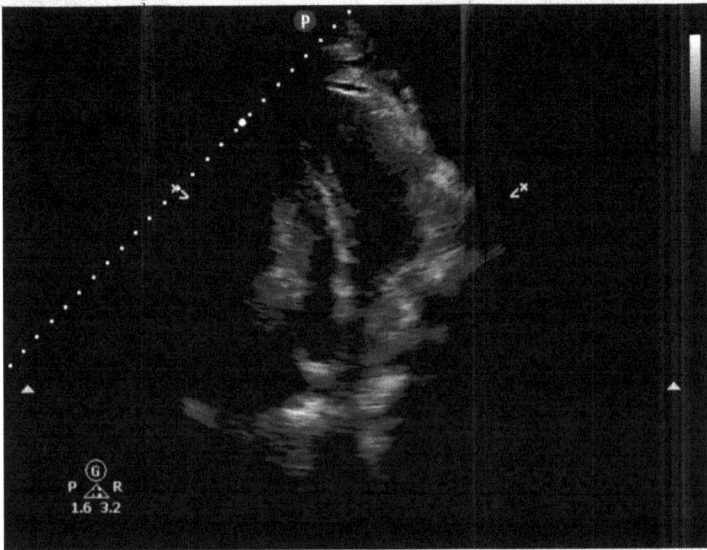

Figure 7.3

Apical-four-chamber view of the heart revealing a large pericardial effusion with echocardiographic signs of cardiac tamponade

The bedside echocardiograms (Fig. 7.1, 7.2, 7.3) reveal a large circumscribed pericardial effusion with hemodynamic compromise and pericardial tamponade, including right atrial systolic collapse and right ventricular diastolic collapse. In addition, a scan of the IVC (not shown) was found to be plethoric with minimal respirophasic variation, consistent with the patient's presentation of obstructive shock.

A pericardial effusion appears as an anechoic stripe adjacent to the pericardium, which is usually circumferential, and should extend anterior to the descending aorta (visualized posterior to the left atrium on a parasternal long axis view) [3].

> **Pitfall:** If a loculated pericardial effusion is present, as is the case with this patient, it may not be evident on all views and may be missed if multiple views are not obtained. This reinforces the importance of obtaining multiple views when performing a bedside echocardiogram.

> **Pitfall:** A pleural effusion can be mistakenly identified as a pericardial effusion. In contrast to pericardial effusions, pleural effusions will collect posterior to the descending aorta. The following image, of a different patient with both pericardial and pleural effusions, illustrates this concept (Fig. 7.4).

> **Pitfall:** Epicardial fat pad can be mistaken as a pericardial effusion. An epicardial fat pad will usually be located only anteriorly (not circumferentially), and is not completely anechoic.

ULTRASOUND IMAGE QUALITY ASSURANCE

An important aspect of ultrasound is appropriate and optimal image acquisition. The bedside echocardiograms show optimal gain and depth. The provider appropriately captures several views. While a small pericardial effusion may be noted in the apical 4-chamber and parasternal long views, the loculated effusion in this particular patient is only really marked in the parasternal short axis! This highlights the importance of obtaining multiple views when performing an echocardiogram, and a general rule to follow for all ultrasounds you perform.

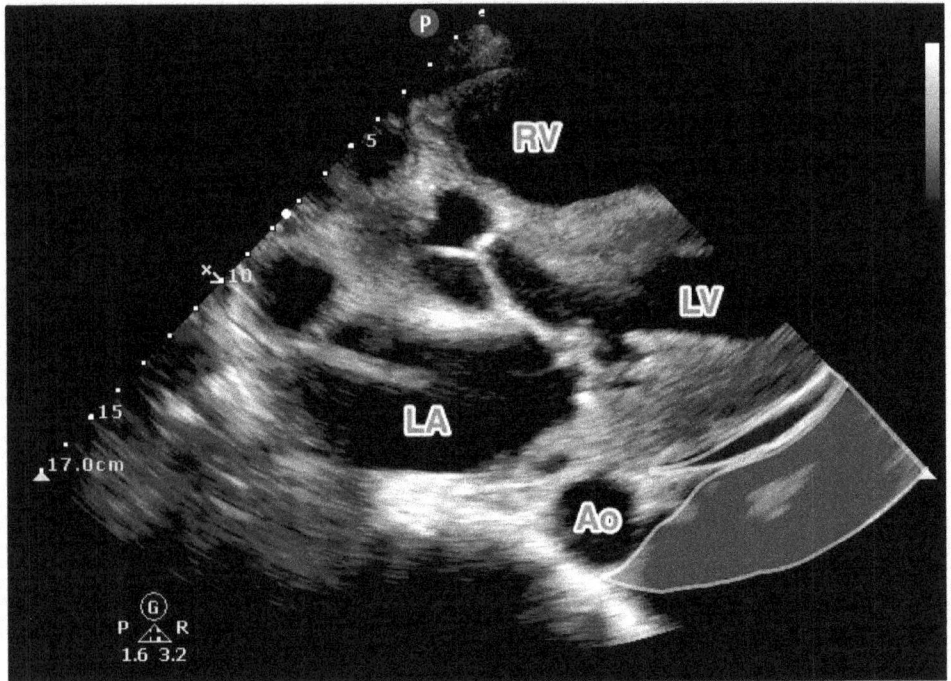

Figure 7.4

Parasternal long axis view of the heart showing a pericardial effusion anterior to the descending thoracic aorta (Ao), whereas a pleural effusion is seen posterior to the aorta. LA=left atrium, RV=right ventricle, LV=left ventricle

DISPOSITION AND CASE CONCLUSION

Patients who present to the ED with shock require expeditious care and treatment. The use of bedside ultrasound is critical in narrowing the differential diagnosis and providing prompt, high-quality patient care. This case highlights the role of resuscitative ultrasound in guiding the clinical pathway and management of the patient.

In this case, the cardiac catheterization lab was activated for emergent pericardiocentesis within minutes of obtaining the bedside echocardiogram. A formal echocardiogram obtained in the cardiac suite confirmed the initial focused echocardiogram findings of a loculated anterior pericardial effusion. Due to the loculated nature of this effusion, the pericardiocentesis was difficult, and the patient was taken emergently to the operating room for a pericardial window, pericardial stripping, and a total pericardiectomy. She was discharged from the hospital 10 days later in good condition. The cause of the initial effusion was thought to be lupus related.

While bedside echocardiography can accurately visualize pericardial effusions, it is important to remember that this does not necessarily mean the patient has cardiac tamponade. Furthermore, the size of a pericardial effusion does not predict tamponade or hemodynamic instability; a large effusion may be chronic and the patient may be asymptomatic, and a small effusion may cause tamponade and hemodynamic instability.

Cardiac tamponade

Echocardiographic signs of tamponade or impending tamponade include:

- Right atrial (RA) collapse in systole,
- Right ventricular (RV) collapse in diastole, and/or
- Visualization of a plethoric IVC with minimal respirophasic variability [4]

This can be fairly easily obtained and visualized with M-mode (which represents the motion of structures over time) in a parasternal long axis view of the heart with the M-line transecting through both the RV and mitral valve. For further discussion on this as well as a great image, refer to an excellent article by Nagdev and Stone [4].

While a plethoric IVC is non-specific and can be seen in other scenarios such as fluid overload, pulmonary embolism, and right heart strain, it can be helpful in diagnosing cardiac tamponade in the right clinical context.

TAKE-HOME POINTS

1. The use of resuscitative bedside ultrasound is critical in guiding care in patients with shock.

2. Be aware of common pitfalls when assessing for pericardial effusions:

   • Mistaking a fat pad or pleural effusion as a pericardial effusion
   • Missing a localized, loculated pericardial effusion

3. Not all pericardial effusions cause cardiac tamponade.

4. Echocardiographic evidence of cardiac tamponade includes right atrial collapse during systole, right ventricular collapse during diastole, and a plethoric IVC with decreased respirophasic variation.

REFERENCES

1. Ghane MR, Gharib M, Ebrahimi A, Saeedi M, Akbari-Kamrani M, Rezaee M, Rasouli H. Accuracy of early rapid ultrasound in shock (RUSH) examination performed by emergency physician for diagnosis of shock etiology in critically ill patients. J Emerg Trauma Shock. 2015 Jan-Mar;8(1):5-10. PMID: 25709245.

2. Atkinson PR, McAuley DJ, Kendall RJ, Abeyakoon O, Reid CG, Connolly J, Lewis D. Abdominal and Cardiac Evaluation with Sonography in Shock (ACES): an approach by emergency physicians for the use of ultrasound in patients with undifferentiated hypotension. Emerg Med J. 2009 Feb;26(2): 87-91. PMID 19164614.

3. Goodman A, Perera P, Mailhot T, Mandavia D. The role of bedside ultrasound in the diagnosis of pericardial effusion and cardiac tamponade. J Emerg Trauma Shock. 2012 Jan;5(1):72-5. PMID: 22416160.

4. Nagdev A, Stone MB. Point-of-care ultrasound evaluation of pericardial effusions: does this patient have cardiac tamponade? Resuscitation 2011; 82(6): 671-3. PMID: 21397379.

46F with Right-Sided Abdominal and Flank Pain

OBJECTIVES

1. Describe the role of ultrasound in patients who present with suspected renal colic.
2. Summarize the major findings of the 2014 study by Smith-Bindman et al. and the significance of imaging modality selection for patients with suspected renal colic.
3. Identify and describe the differences between mild, moderate, and severe hydronephrosis on ultrasound.
4. Recognize the utility of color Doppler in renal ultrasound.

CASE PRESENTATION

An otherwise healthy 46-year-old female presents to the ED with 6 hours of right-sided abdominal pain. She complains of pain in the right lower quadrant (RLQ) of the abdomen, radiating to the right flank. She is noted to be febrile, but appears well. Review of systems is positive for dysuria, but she denies nausea, vomiting, diarrhea, or vaginal discharge or bleeding. She denies any history of abdominal surgeries. On examination, she has abdominal tenderness to palpation in the RLQ without rebound or guarding and no costovertebral angle tenderness.

VITAL SIGNS

BP	123/65 mmHg
P	87 bpm
RR	20 breaths/min
O2	100% room air
T	38.7°C

DIFFERENTIAL DIAGNOSIS
Appendicitis
Ectopic pregnancy
Gastroenteritis
Nephrolithiasis
Ovarian torsion
Pyelonephritis
Urinary tract infection

INITIAL WORKUP

The patient's lab results were significant for a leukocytosis (WBC 18.8/hpf), and a negative pregnancy test. An abdominopelvis computed tomography (CT) scan with intravenous contrast was ordered to rule-out appendicitis. A urinalysis was positive for leukocytes, small blood, > 100 WBC/hpf, and many bacteria. At this point in the patient's workup, it was change of shift and the patient was signed out as "follow-up CT to rule out appendicitis; if negative, treat for pyelonephritis." The oncoming provider, upon re-evaluating the patient, performed a point-of-care focused renal ultrasound.

POINT-OF-CARE ULTRASOUND was performed which showed the following:

Figure 8.1

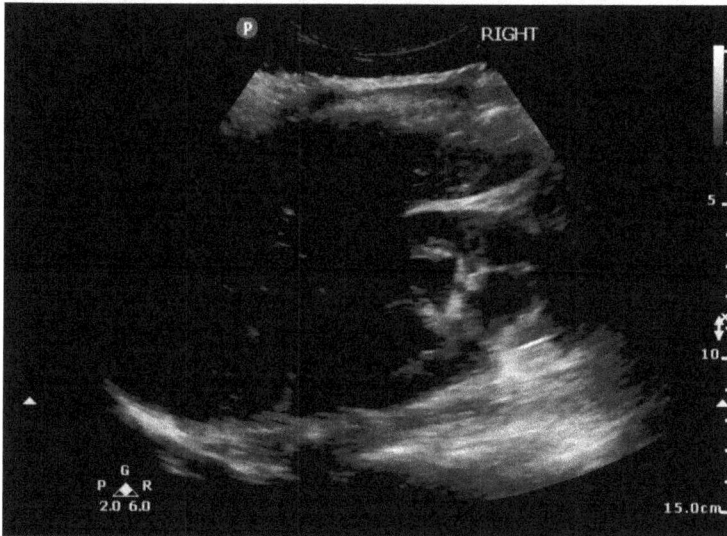

Ultrasound of the right kidney reveals moderate hydronephrosis

Figure 8.2

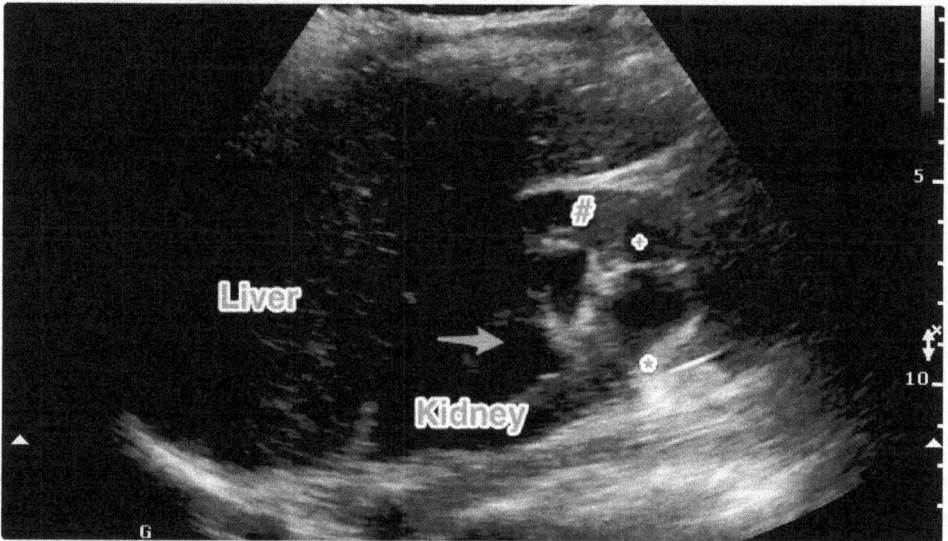

Image from Figure 8.1 showing the right kidney with moderate hydronephrosis (arrow). Renal cortex (#), medullary pyramid (+), and renal sinus (*) are also identified.

Figure 8.3

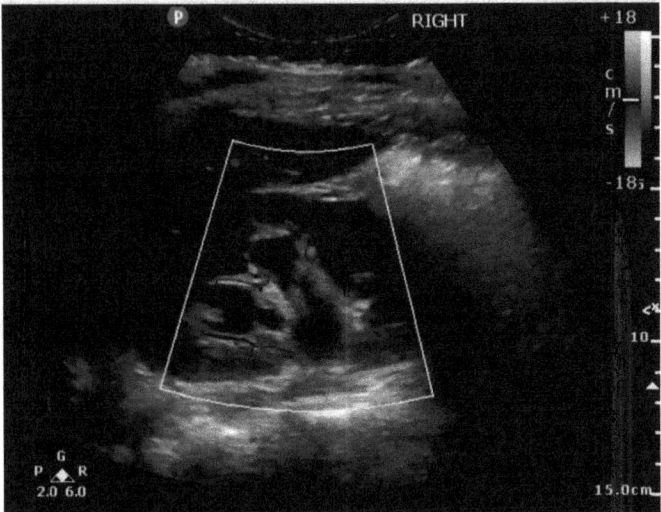

Right kidney showing no color Doppler flow in anechoic areas consistent with hydronephrosis

Figure 8.4

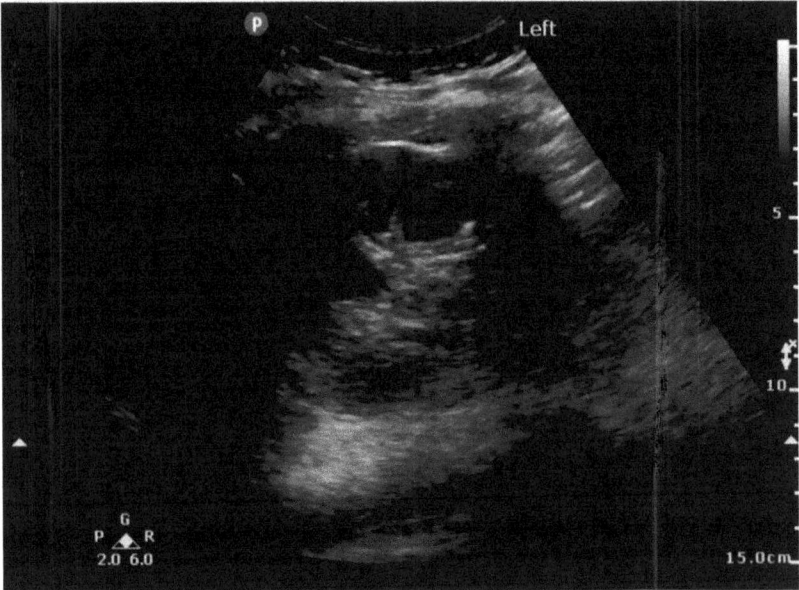

Normal left kidney with no evidence of hydronephrosis

ULTRASOUND IMAGE QUALITY ASSURANCE

The images obtained (Fig. 8.1, 8.2, 8.3, 8.4) show the standard views that should be obtained when performing a focused point-of-care renal study. A curvilinear probe is used and positioned in a coronal plane. These views should be very familiar to emergency physicians, as they are similar to the right upper quadrant (RUQ) and left upper quadrant (LUQ) views of a FAST exam. Both kidneys are scanned fully in both planes, using the liver and spleen as acoustic windows.

The primary indication for performing a focused bedside renal study in the ED is to look for hydronephrosis, which is classified into one of three grades – mild, moderate, or severe. Mild hydronephrosis appears as a dilation of the renal pelvis (Fig. 8.5), moderate hydronephrosis as a dilation of the renal pelvis and calyces (Fig. 8.6), and severe hydronephrosis as a ballooning of the calyces and thinning of the renal cortex (Fig. 8.7) [1].

Figure 8.5

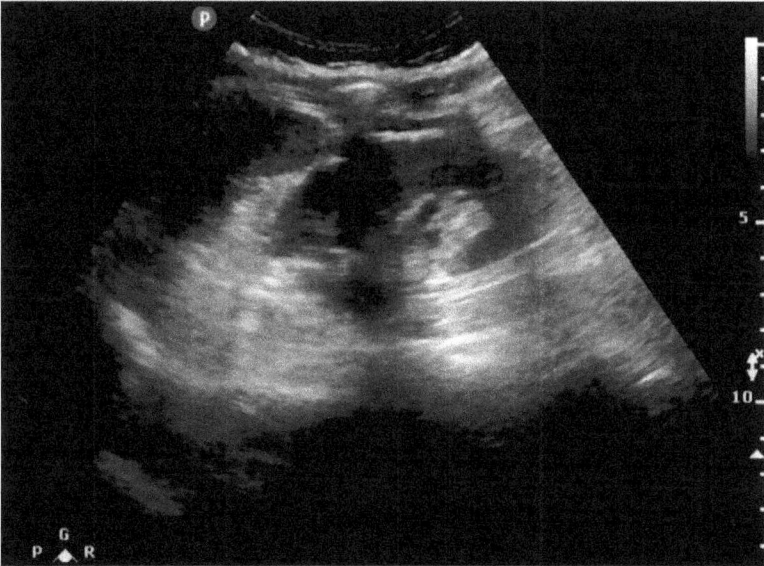

Grading of hydronephrosis: MILD

Figure 8.6

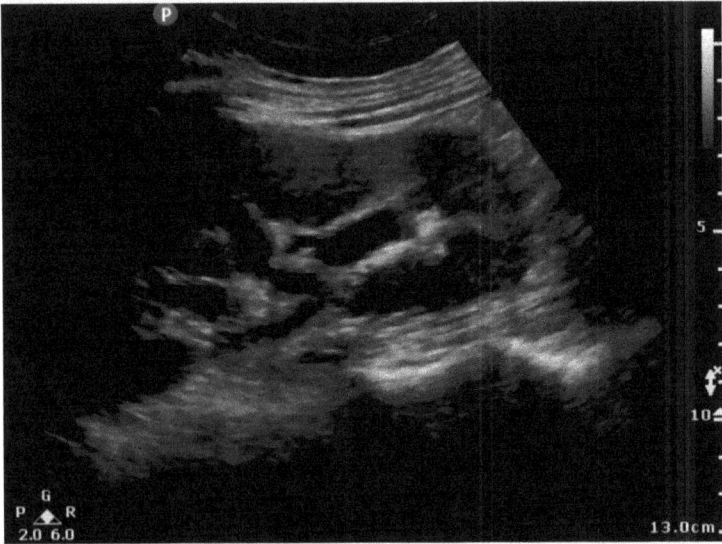

Grading of hydronephrosis: MODERATE

Figure 8.7

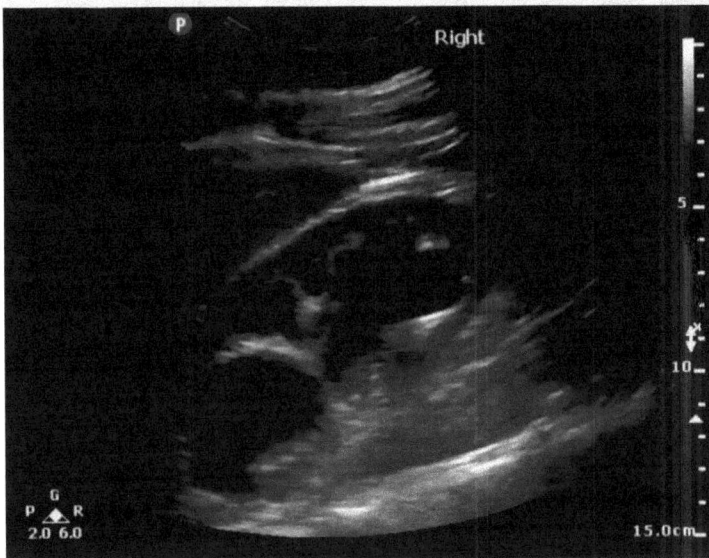

Grading of hydronephrosis: SEVERE

Pitfall: Normal renal vasculature is often mistaken for hydronephrosis, because both appear anechoic (black) on a B-mode or grayscale clip (Fig. 8.8). Placing color Doppler over the area will help to distinguish these from one another (Fig. 8.9). Renal vasculature will demonstrate flow with color Doppler, whereas hydronephrosis will remain anechoic without flow.

Figure 8.8

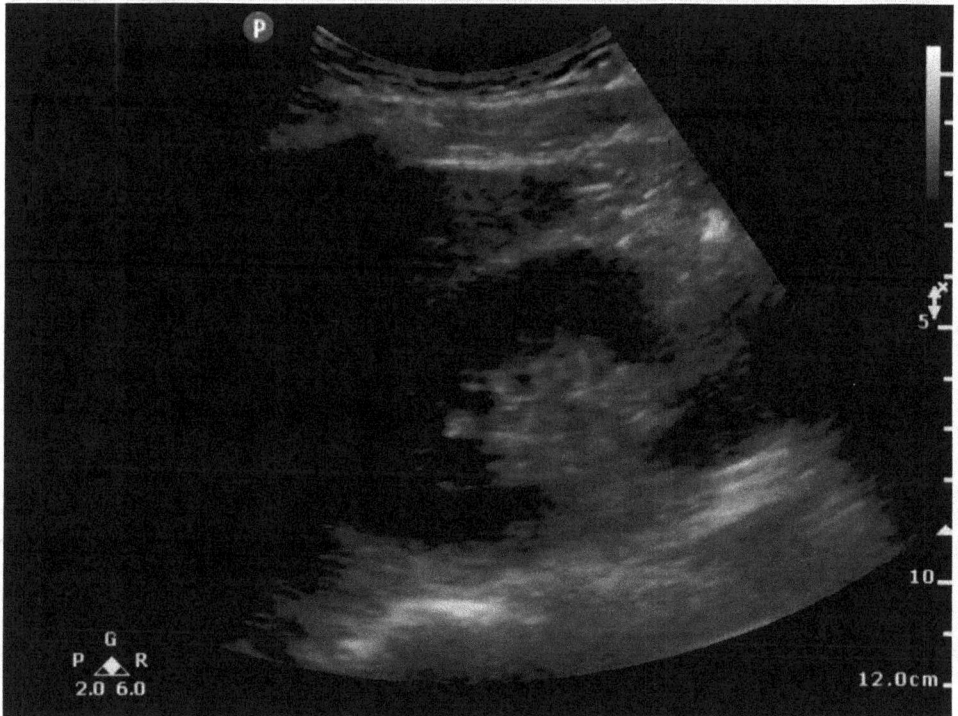

Right kidney with anechoic areas, which is hard to distinguish between mild hydronephrosis versus normal renal vasculature, without using color Doppler

Figure 8.9

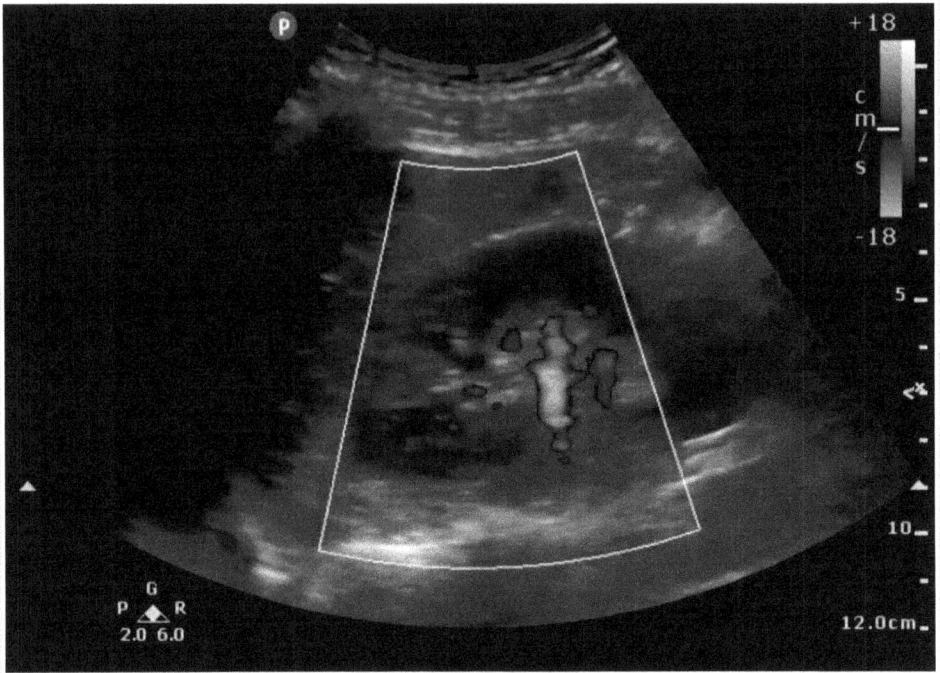

Color Doppler imaging of the same right kidney from Figure 8.8, showing that the anechoic areas have color flow and thus indicative of renal vasculature rather than hydronephrosis.

DISPOSITION AND CASE CONCLUSION

Given the findings of moderate right-sided hydronephrosis on the point-of-care ultrasound, the CT order was changed from a contrast study to a non-contrast flank CT study, given the concern for an obstructed and infected kidney stone.

The CT abdomen and pelvis revealed a large, 7.37 mm obstructing renal calculus in the right mid-ureter with upstream moderate hydroureteronephrosis and perinephric stranding due to infectious or inflammatory etiology (Fig. 8.10).

The patient was given IV antibiotics, and urology was consulted. She was taken to the operating room for cystoscopy and right ureteral stent placement for urgent decompression. On post-operative day 3, the patient was discharged home in stable condition, afebrile, and with her pain well controlled.

Patients presenting to the ED with flank or kidney pain account for over 2 million annual ED visits in the US [1]. CT is often the initial imaging study of choice given its high sensitivity (97%) and specificity (96%) for diagnosing nephrolithiasis [2]. However, there has been a concerning 10-fold increase in the use of CT for diagnosis of kidney stones over the past 15 years, with no change in frequency of diagnosis or hospital admissions [3].

Figure 8.7

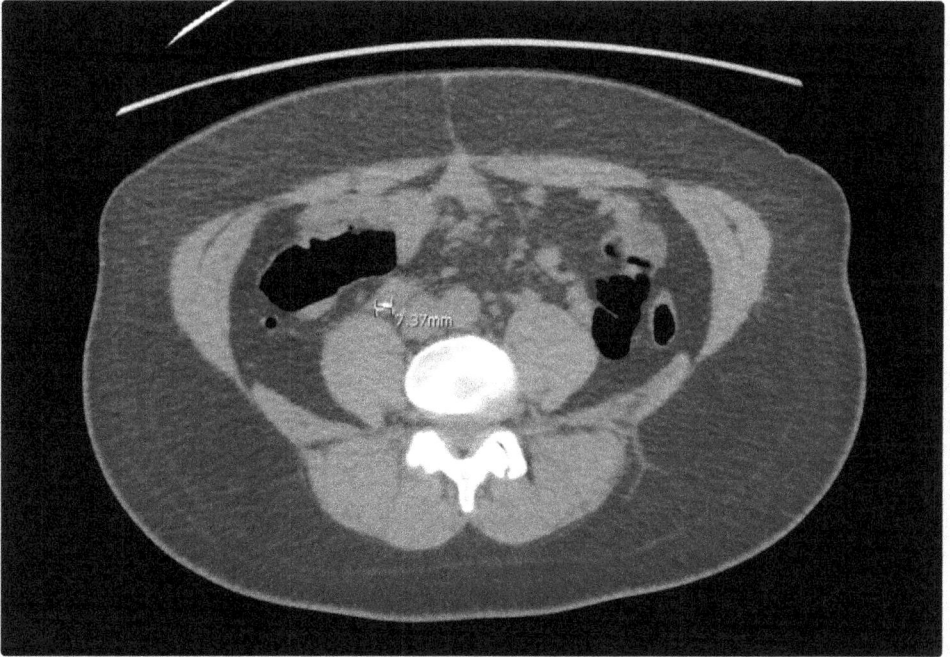

Non-contrast abdominopelvis CT showing a 7.37 mm renal calculus in the right mid-ureter

Point-of-care renal ultrasound can play a vital role in the diagnosis and management of patients who present to the ED with abdominal or flank pain. The primary indication for renal ultrasound in the ED is to assess for hydronephrosis, an indirect sign of ureteral obstruction. Although ultrasound is poorly sensitive for directly imaging stones, one study revealed that resulting hydronephrosis may be easier to identify in patients with larger stones (90% sensitivity for detecting hydronephrosis with stones >6 mm, compared with 75% sensitivity with stones <6 mm) [4]. This can be reassuring in the clinical setting of uncomplicated ureterolithiasis, as smaller stones are likely to pass on their own without intervention, and "missing" hydronephrosis with these smaller stones is unlikely to change clinical outcomes.

A large multicenter study published in 2014 in the *New England Journal of Medicine* found that ultrasonography should be used as the initial imaging modality for patients with suspected nephrolithiasis, with further imaging studies performed based on the findings and discretion of the clinician [5]. Patients enrolled in the study were randomized to one of three initial imaging modalities:

1. Point-of-care ultrasonography by an emergency physician
2. Radiology-performed ultrasonography
3. CT

Comparison of the three groups at 30 days showed no statistically significant difference in high-risk diagnoses with complications, serious adverse events, pain control, return ED visits, hospitalizations, or diagnostic accuracy [5].

In this patient case, the point-of-care ultrasound and clinical picture suggested a diagnosis of complicated ureterolithiasis (i.e. a potentially obstructed and infected kidney stone requiring urologic intervention), and thus a CT was rightfully obtained.

TAKE-HOME POINTS

1. Consider ultrasonography instead of CT as the initial imaging modality in patients who present with a strong suspicion for nephrolithiasis, especially in younger and female patients.

2. Although CT has a higher sensitivity for kidney stones than ultrasonography, this increased sensitivity does not necessarily improve diagnostic accuracy or decrease serious adverse events [5].

3. Point-of-care ultrasonography by emergency physicians for identifying hydronephrosis has a moderate sensitivity (72.6%) and specificity (73.3%), with much higher sensitivity (92.7%) in those with additional ultrasound fellowship training [1].

4. The use of color Doppler can help distinguish hydronephrosis from normal renal vasculature.

REFERENCES

1. Herbst MK, Rosenberg G, Daniels B, Gross CP, Singh D, Molinaro AM, Luty S, Moore CL. Effect of provider experience on clinician-performed ultrasonography for hydronephrosis in patients with suspected renal colic. Ann Emerg Med. 2014 Sep;64(3):269-76. PMID: 24630203.

2. Dalziel PJ, Noble VE. Bedside ultrasound and the assessment of renal colic: a review. Emerg Med J. 2013 Jan;30(1):3-8. PMID: 22685250.

3. Moore CL, Scoutt L. Sonography first for acute flank pain? J Ultrasound Med. 2012 Nov;31(11):1703-11. PMID: 23091240.

4. Riddell J, Case A, Wopat R, Beckham S, Lucas M, McClung CD, Swadron S. Sensitivity of emergency bedside ultrasound to detect hydronephrosis in patients with computed tomography-proven stones. West J Emerg Med. 2014 Feb;15(1):96-100. PMID: 24578772.

5. Smith-Bindman R, Aubin C, Bailitz J, Bengiamin RN, Camargo CA Jr, Corbo J, Dean AJ, Goldstein RB, Griffey RT, Jay GD, Kang TL, Kriesel DR, Ma OJ, Mallin M, Manson W, Melnikow J, Miglioretti DL, Miller SK, Mills LD, Miner JR, Moghadassi M, Noble VE, Press GM, Stoller ML, Valencia VE, Wang J, Wang RC, Cummings SR. Ultrasonography versus computed tomography for suspected nephrolithiasis. N Engl J Med. 2014 Sep 18;371(12):1100-10. PMID: 25229916.

76M with Right-Sided Vision Loss

OBJECTIVES

1. Explain the utility of ultrasound in the diagnosis of retinal detachment.
2. Describe the sonographic findings of retinal detachment.
3. List the potential pitfalls of ocular ultrasound.
4. Summarize the sensitivity and specificity of point-of-care ultrasound by emergency physicians in the diagnosis of retinal detachment.

CASE PRESENTATION

A 76-year-old man with hypertension presents to the ED with 5 hours of sudden onset, right-sided vision loss. He notes seeing flashes of light in the periphery of his field of vision followed by several "floaters". He denies any trauma, headache, or pain. On physical examination, he appears well and is in no acute distress. His neurologic examination is unremarkable. His pupils are 3 mm, round, and reactive to light bilaterally. His visual acuity is 20/20 OS, and 20/100 OD. His intraocular pressures are measured at 8 mmHg bilaterally.

VITAL SIGNS

BP	131/62 mmHg
P	78 bpm
RR	20 breaths/min
O2	99% room air
T	37.4°C

DIFFERENTIAL DIAGNOSIS

Migraine
Optic neuropathy
Posterior vitreous detachment
Retinal artery/vein occlusion
Retinal detachment
Stroke/Transient ischemic attack
Uveitis

POINT-OF-CARE ULTRASOUND was performed which showed the following:

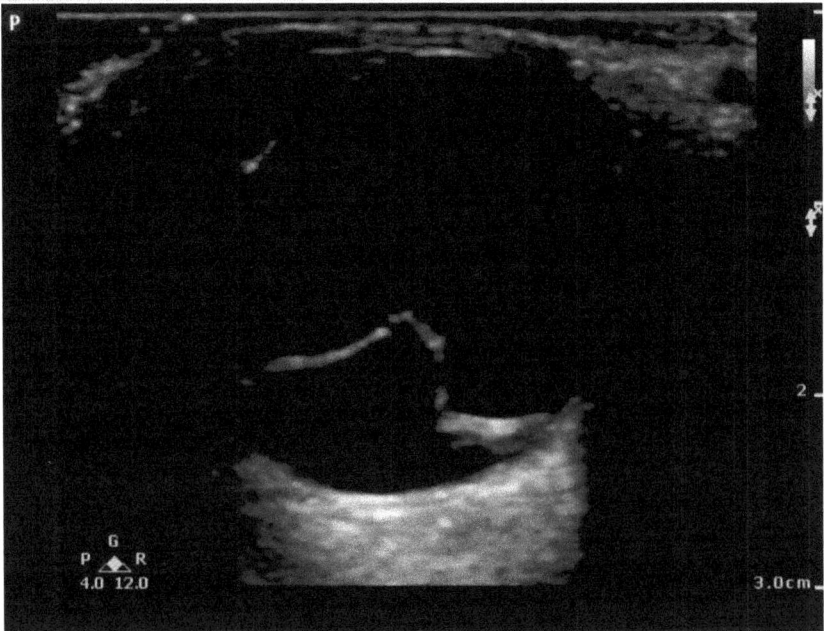

Figure 9.1

Retinal detachment of the affected eye

ULTRASOUND IMAGE QUALITY ASSURANCE

The eye, being a superficial fluid-filled structure, is an optimal organ for diagnostic ultrasonography. Point-of-care ocular ultrasound is fairly straightforward. Images are obtained using a high-frequency linear transducer with the "ocular" setting on the ultrasound machine, if available.

Figure 9.2

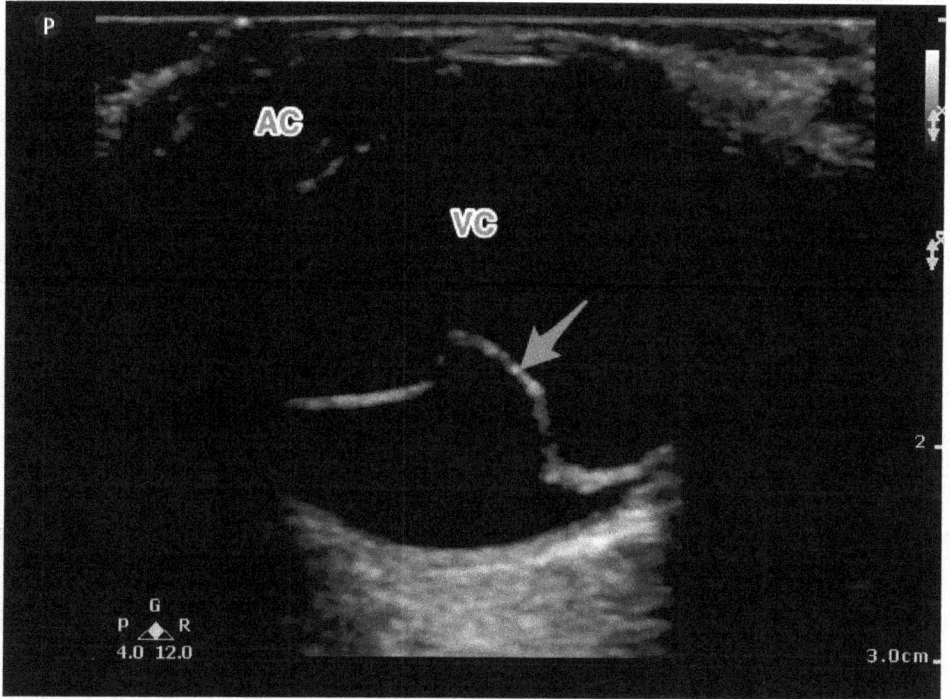

Ocular ultrasound showing a retinal detachment (arrow). Also note the anterior chamber (AC) and vitreous chamber (VC).

A retinal detachment (RD) is a separation of the two layers of the retina, which invariably causes blindness if left untreated [1]. On ultrasound, this appears as a bright hyperechoic wavy line within the vitreous chamber peeling off the posterior aspect of the eye (Fig. 9.1, 9.2). Associated vitreous hemorrhage may also be visualized as hyperechoic strands within the vitreous chamber that move with eye movement, and has the appearance of clothes tumbling in a washing machine (The "Washing Machine Sign").

To perform an ocular ultrasound, apply a generous amount of gel over a closed eyelid, with or without a tegaderm. Both the affected and unaffected eye should be examined for comparison, with normal landmarks and anatomy noted (Fig. 9.3).

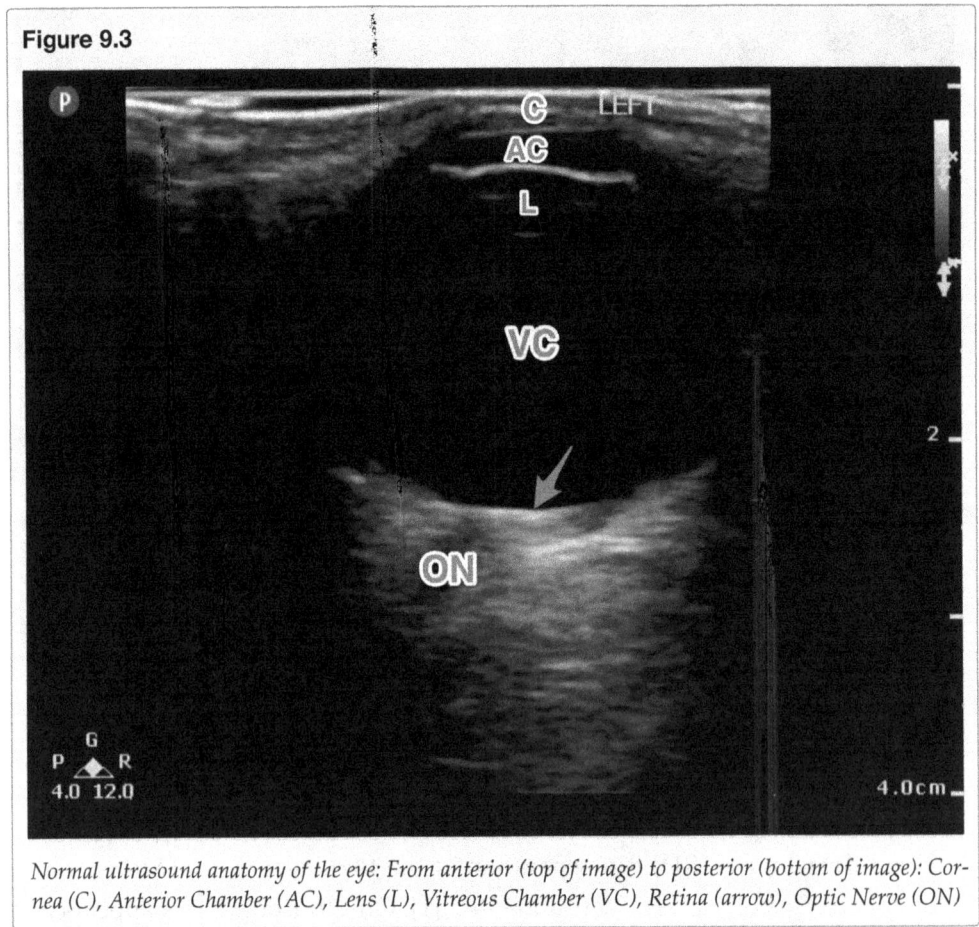

Figure 9.3

Normal ultrasound anatomy of the eye: From anterior (top of image) to posterior (bottom of image): Cornea (C), Anterior Chamber (AC), Lens (L), Vitreous Chamber (VC), Retina (arrow), Optic Nerve (ON)

It is especially important to optimize the gain, or brightness, with ocular studies. Generally, the gain is set slightly higher than usual to just the point of visualizing small echogenic material within the vitreous chamber. This avoids missing a potential subtle RD if the gain is set too low. With the ultrasound probe oriented transversely then longitudinally over the globe, the probe is fanned back and forth, spanning the entire globe. Finally, the patient should move their eye in all directions in order to fully evaluate the entire globe for pathology.

Common Pitfalls in Ocular Ultrasound:

1. **Inadequate gain:** Gain, or brightness, that is set too low can miss subtle structures including a detached retinal flap. Gain that is too high can increase acoustic enhancement artifacts posteriorly, also with the risk of missing a RD.
2. **Artifacts:** It can be normal to see artifacts within the vitreous chamber, which may appear as bright echogenic material. Movement of the eye should cause artifacts to "disappear". (Fig. 9.4, 9.5)

Figure 9.4

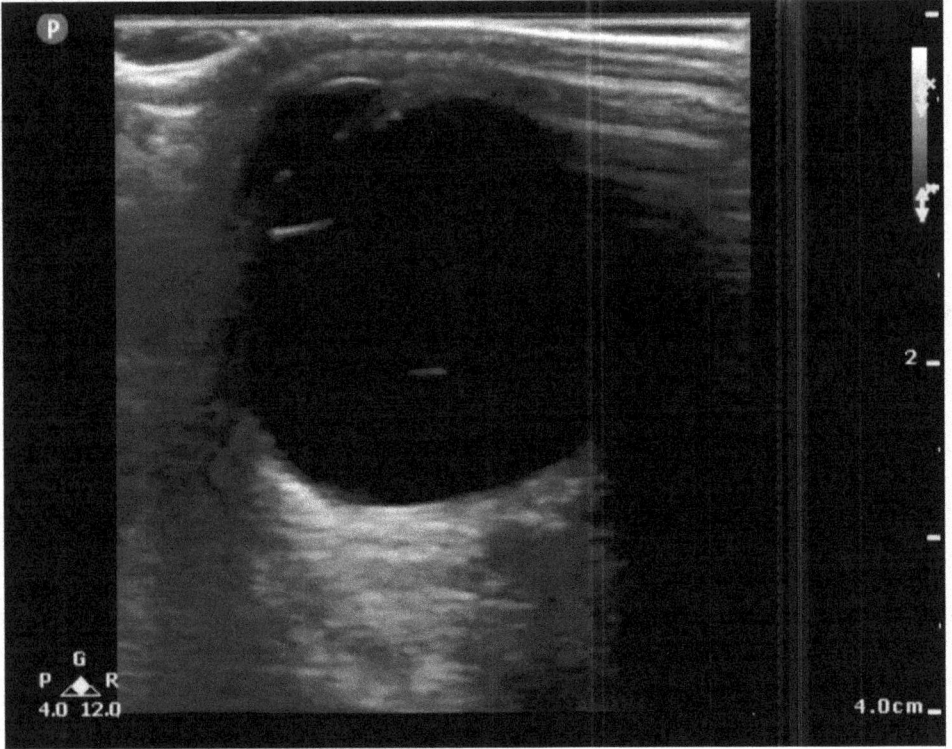

Normal ocular ultrasound with artifact in the vitreous chamber

Figure 9.5

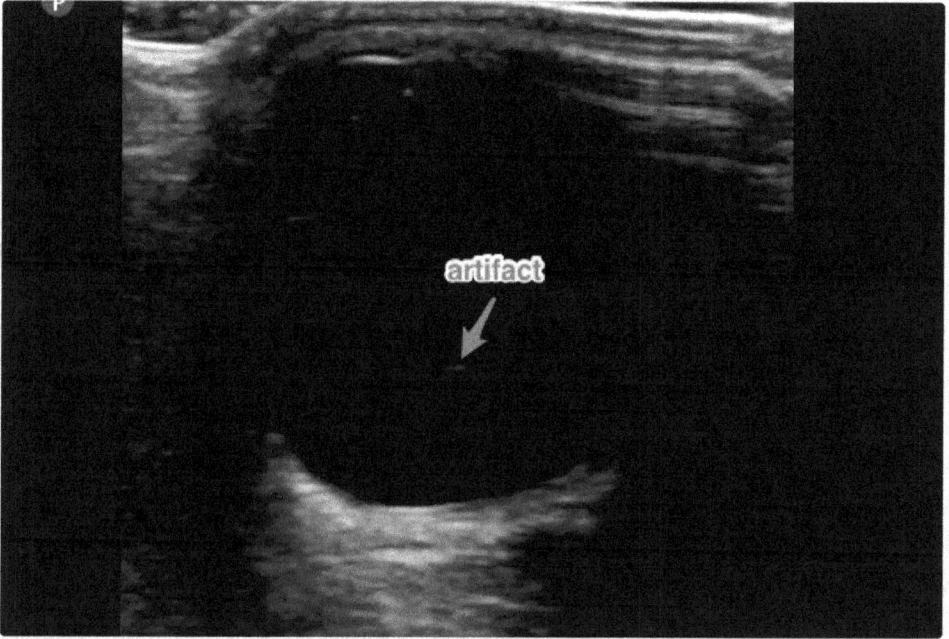

Image from Figure 9.4 labelling the artifact finding, which sometimes can be mistaken for retinal detachment or other pathology.

ULTRASOUND FANATIC SIDE NOTE:

Ophthalmologists were among the first physicians to use ultrasound in their clinical practice. Ultrasound of the orbit has been described in the ophthalmology literature to aid in the diagnosis of retinal detachment as early as 1957 by Oksala and Lehtinen [2]. Their use of A (Amplitude)-mode, visualized as a graph of spikes along an axis, differs from the more conventional B (Brightness)-mode, the series of 2D images that we currently use in the ED. For additional reading, please refer to History of Ophthalmic Ultrasound by Lizzi and Coleman [3].

DISPOSITION AND CASE CONCLUSION

Given the concerning finding for a RD on ultrasound, ophthalmology was consulted and confirmed the diagnosis. The patient underwent definitive treatment and his visual acuity was fortunately preserved.

Retinal detachment affects 1 in 300 people, and remains a time-critical and vision-threatening diagnosis that ED providers must consider in patients presenting with ocular complaints [4]. Patients presenting with RD typically complain of sudden-onset unilateral painless loss of vision or visual field deficits. They may describe "flashing lights", "floaters", or "spider webs" in their field of vision. If the macula is not detached, the goal is to undergo definitive treatment to preserve the macula. Time to treatment is critical in these cases as the duration of macular detachment is inversely related to a patient's ultimate visual acuity [5]. Patients will often have good outcomes if treated promptly. Thus, a high-level of suspicion and ophthalmologic consultation with close follow-up is warranted for definitive care.

The vast range of ocular pathologies that present to the ED is a diagnostic challenging without a dedicated fundoscopic examination. Unfortunately, non-dilated direct fundoscopy is often inadequate, and has been shown to miss 38% of retinal pathologies that required intervention [6]. The use of point-of-care ultrasound serves as a vital adjunct to clinical assessment in the time-critical diagnosis of intraocular diseases including RD. While seemingly an "advanced" ultrasound technique, the findings of RD are not subtle and can be easily identified, as was seen in this particular case. In fact, a prospective study by Shinar et al. found that emergency physicians can accurately diagnose RD using bedside ultrasound with a sensitivity of 97% and specificity of 92% [7]. Additionally, Blaivas et al. showed that 60 out of 61 intraocular diseases were accurately diagnosed by the emergency physician with bedside ultrasound when using an ophthalmologists' evaluation as the gold standard [8].

The main indications for ocular ultrasound in the ED expand beyond looking for RD, and include assessing for vitreous hemorrhage, intraocular foreign bodies, lens dislocation, and signs of elevated intracranial pressure (Table 9.1). Note that the only absolute contraindication to ocular ultrasound is a suspected ruptured globe, in which case no pressure should be placed on the globe.

INDICATIONS FOR OCULAR ULTRASOUND
Acute vision changes or loss of vision
Orbital trauma (when globe rupture is not suspected)
Atraumatic eye pain
Elevated intracranial pressure
Intraocular foreign body

CONTRAINDICATIONS TO OCULAR ULTRASOUND
Suspected globe rupture

Table 9.1. *Indications and contraindications for ocular ultrasound in the Emergency Department*

TAKE-HOME POINTS

1. A retinal detachment (RD) is a time-sensitive ophthalmologic emergency that invariably leads to blindness if left untreated. If there is a suspicion of a RD, ophthalmology consultation is warranted.

2. While a dilated fundoscopic exam is typically required for diagnosis of RD, this is often not feasible or available in a busy ED or community setting.

3. Emergency physicians are highly accurate in the diagnosis of intraocular pathologies including RD with the aid of point-of-care ultrasound with 97% sensitivity and 92% specificity [8].

REFERENCES

1. Bhatia K, Sharma R. Eye emergencies. In: Adams JG. Emergency medicine. Philadelphia: Saunders Elsevier; 2008. 213–32.

2. Oksala A, Lehtinen A. Diagnostics of detachment of the retina by means of ultrasound. Acta Ophthalmol (Copenh). 1957;35(5):461-7.PMID: 13497646.

3. Lizzi FL, Coleman DJ. History of ophthalmic ultrasound. J Ultrasound Med. 2004 Oct;23(10):1255-66. PMID: 15448314.

4. Schott ML, Pierog JE, Williams SR. Pitfalls in the use of ocular ultrasound for evaluation of acute vision loss. J Emerg Med. 2013; 44(6): 1136-9. PMID: 23522956.

5. Marx et al. Rosen's Emergency Medicine: Concepts and Clinical Practice, 8th ed; 2014.

6. Siegel BS, Thompson AK, Yolton DP, Reinke AR, Yolton RL. A comparison of diagnostic outcomes with and without pupillary dilatation. J Am Optom Assoc. 1990; 61(1): 25-34. PMID: 2319090.

7. Shinar Z, Chan L, Orlinsky M. Use of ocular ultrasound for the evaluation of retinal detachment. J Emerg Med. 2011; 40(1): 53-7. PMID: 19625159.

8. Blaivas M, Theodoro D, Sierzenski PR. A study of bedside ocular ultrasonography in the emergency department. Acad Emerg Med. 2002; 9(8): 791-9. PMID: 12153883.

74F with Right Arm Tingling

OBJECTIVES

1. Describe the sonographic findings of an arterial thrombus.
2. Define Angle of Insonation and its effect on performing a vascular study.
3. Identify and describe aliasing and the steps that can be performed to avoid this artifact.

CASE PRESENTATION

A 74-year-old female with atrial fibrillation presents to the ED with 45 minutes of painful right arm tingling that is now resolving. She has been off of warfarin for the past 2 weeks for knee surgery. She reports no right arm weakness or color change. She reports left shoulder pain 12 hours prior to presentation. She has no complaints of shortness of breath or chest pain.

VITAL SIGNS

BP	**L arm**: 150/52 mmHg **R arm**: 30/- mmHg (automatic BP cuff)
P	96 bpm
RR	18 breaths/min
O2	**L arm**: 94% on room air **R arm**: 85% on room air
T	37.3°C

DIFFERENTIAL DIAGNOSIS

Arterial thromboembolism of right arm

Stroke/cerebrovascular accident

Thoracic aortic dissection

PHYSICAL EXAMINATION

Cardiac and Pulmonary
- Normal except for irregularly irregular rhythm

Right Arm
- No palpable radial or brachial pulses
- Normal strength and sensation
- Capillary refill 3 seconds

Left Arm
- Normal radial and brachial pulses
- Normal strength and sensation
- Capillary refill <2 seconds

Lower Extremities
- Normal and symmetric femoral, posterior tibial, and dorsalis pedis pulses bilaterally
- Normal strength and sensation bilaterally

INITIAL WORKUP

The patient's lab results revealed a subtherapeutic INR of 1.5. A CT angiogram of the chest and abdomen was performed due to concern for aortic dissection versus thromboembolism, and revealed:

- No evidence of thoracic aortic dissection
- Normal right brachiocephalic artery seen to axillary artery
- Multiple areas of atherosclerotic disease

Given the ongoing concern for arterial thromboembolic disease, a **POINT-OF-CARE ULTRASOUND** was performed which showed the following:

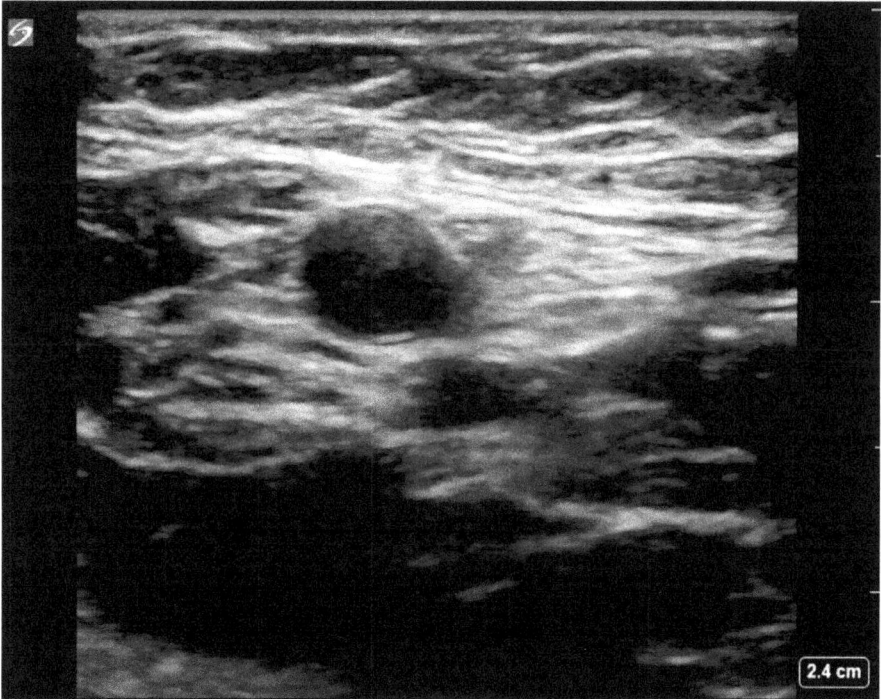

Figure 10.1

2.4 cm

Right axillary artery visualized in B-Mode

Figure 10.2

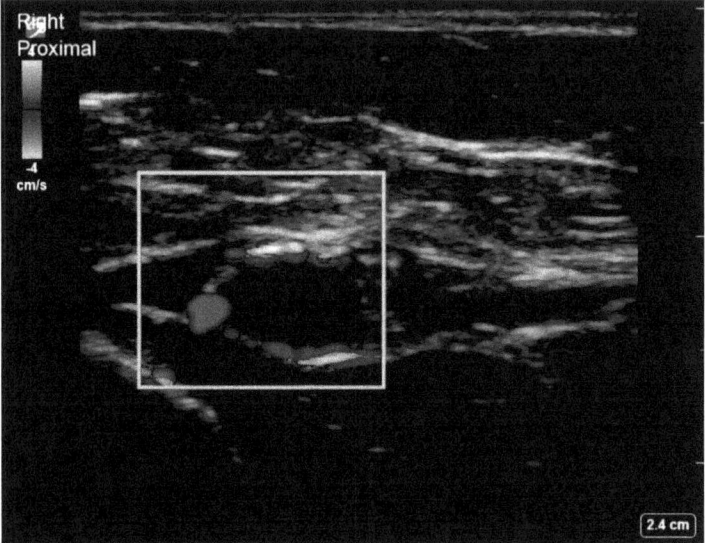

Right axillary artery visualized with color Doppler

Figure 10.3

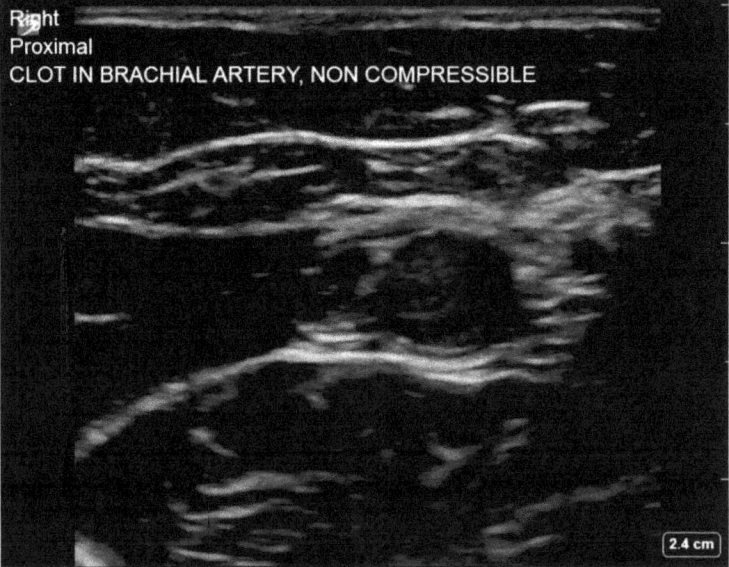

Non-compressible right brachial artery with visualized thrombus

Despite significant external compression with the probe, a visualized thrombus (blue arrow) is seen within a non-compressible brachial artery (Fig. 10.4).

Figure 10.4

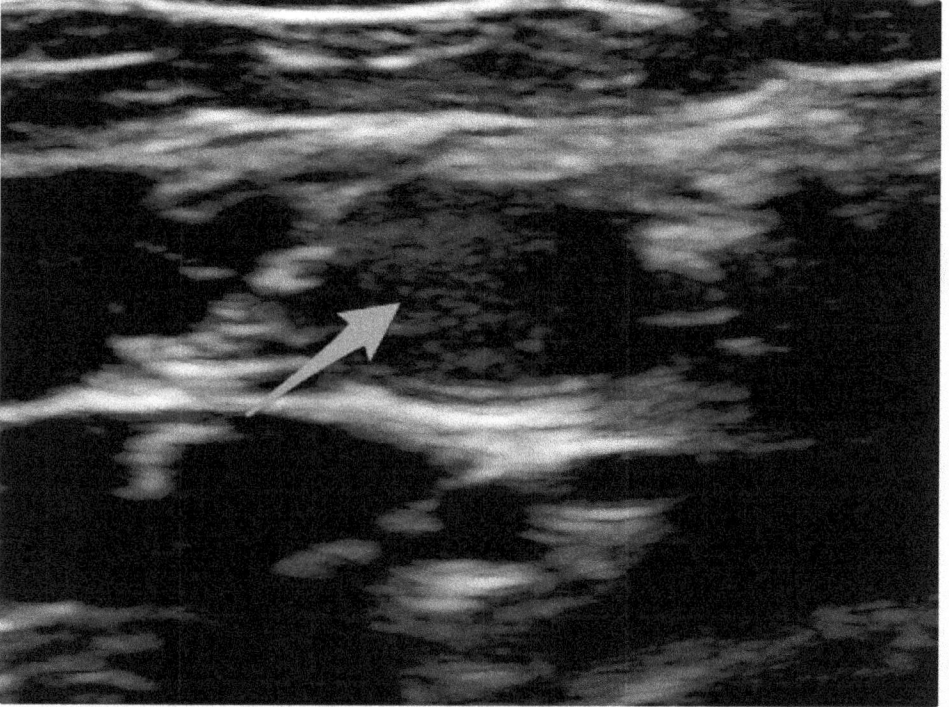

Image from Figure 10.3 demonstrating the intra-arterial thrombus (arrow)
within the right brachial artery

ULTRASOUND IMAGE QUALITY ASSURANCE

Ultrasound evaluation of the vascular system in the extremities is performed using the high-frequency linear transducer. It is important to optimize positioning of the patient when performing any point-of-care ultrasound study; when evaluating the vessels of the upper extremity, the patient should be supine, with the shoulder abducted and externally rotated, and the elbow flexed [1]. Evaluation should include vessel identification, and assessment of vessel compressibility and blood flow. When using B-mode (normal gray scale) the angle of the probe in relation to the vessel should be as close to 90 degrees as possible, which will improve the definition of the vessel as well as the clot. Color Doppler is used to assess direction of flow and can help to differentiate vascular from non-vascular structures such as nerves, lymph nodes, and bursae.

The use of color Doppler is based on measurements of movement. Specifically in this case, it was used to measure the movement of blood in vessels, which is processed as a color flow display. A common misconception is that red is arterial flow, and blue is venous flow; however this is not necessarily always the case. In fact, by default, red is simply indicative of flow moving towards the probe, and blue is indicative of flow moving away from the probe. This is important to note as the Doppler ultrasound beam must be aligned to the direction of flow (angle of insonation), or more parallel to the flow (typically <60 degrees), as opposed to perpendicular to the flow. Figure 10.5 illustrates this concept.

Figure 10.5

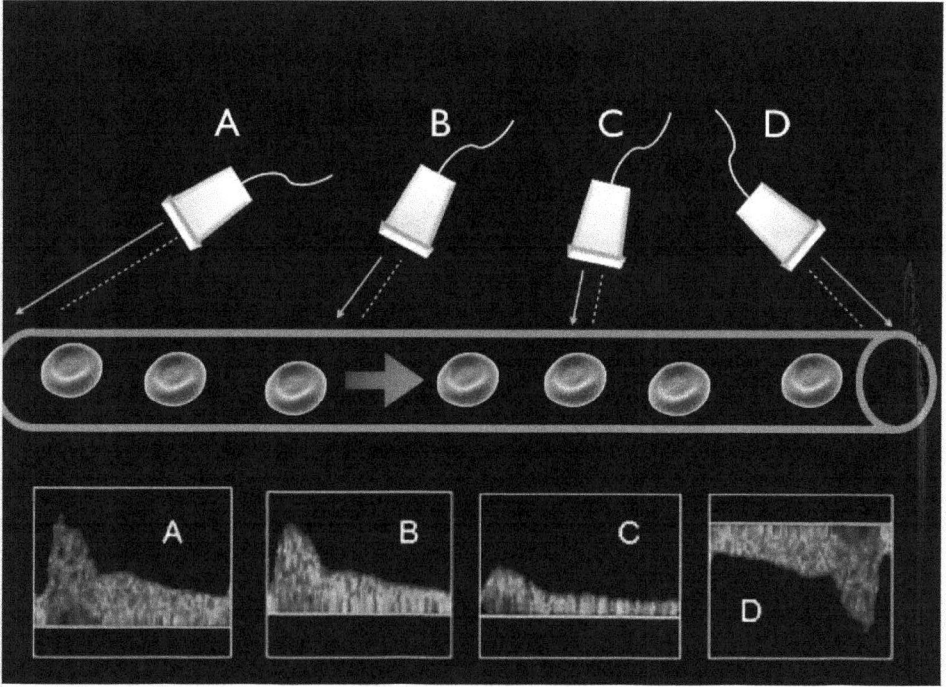

Effect of transducer position (angle of insonation) on color Doppler signal interpretation. Image courtesy of Dr. Mike Mallin.

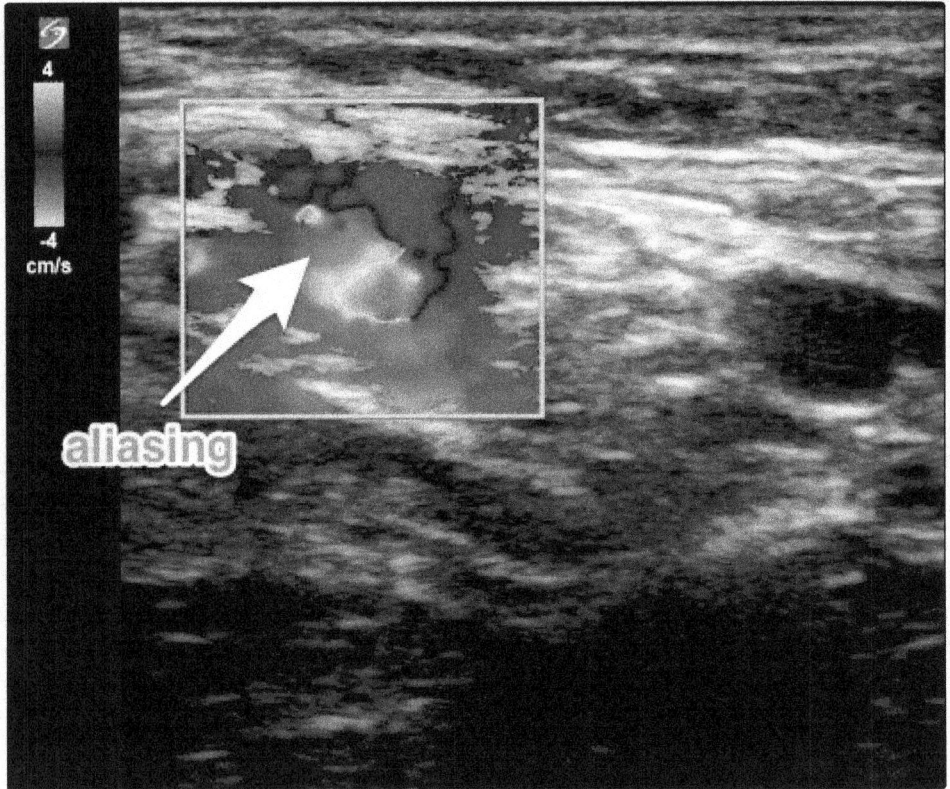

Aliasing artifact seen when the scale is set too low with color Doppler

Also keep in mind your scale when using color Doppler. The higher the flow state (e.g. an artery), the higher your scale should be. If the scale is set too low (as is the case in these clips), you will see more artifact including aliasing, which is an artifact where the color signal "folds over" and falsely appears to be reversing flow (Fig. 10.6). In general when using color and pulsed wave Doppler, the scale should be optimized to minimize aliasing, and the gain should be turned up until color artifact is seen, then turned down just below that point.

Use of a low scale (4 cm/s in this case) on a high-flow vessel can produce an aliasing artifact, falsely appearing as reversal of flow.

DISPOSITION AND CASE CONCLUSION

Given the patient's symptoms and point-of-care ultrasound findings of a non-compressible right brachial artery with visible thrombus, a heparin bolus and infusion were initiated. Vascular surgery was emergently consulted, and the patient was taken for an emergent right brachial artery thrombectomy. Intraoperatively, the surgeons removed a large subacute thrombus with subsequent restoration of normal perfusion in her arm. She was discharged home the next day on enoxaparin as a bridge back to warfarin.

Point-of-care ultrasound for the evaluation of arterial thrombus is an advanced skill, and there is limited evidence on its use by emergency physicians. If there is a concern for arterial thromboembolism in a patient, a vascular surgeon should be consulted given the emergent nature of the process. Revascularization of an ischemic limb within 12 hours has an amputation rate of 6%, and rises to 20% at 24 hours [1]. Given the need for a timely diagnosis, point-of-care ultrasonography can be a beneficial skill for the emergency physician to have, as it can potentially shorten both time-to-diagnosis and time-to-embolectomy.

TAKE-HOME POINTS

1. While there is limited evidence on the use of point-of-care ultrasound by emergency physicians for the detection of acute limb ischemia, classic positive findings of arterial thrombus can decrease time-to-definitive care.

2. Sonographic findings of arterial thromboembolic occlusion include [2]:
   - Non-compressive artery
   - Lack of or altered color Doppler flow in artery
   - Intraluminal echogenic material in artery

3. Optimize your probe position when using color Doppler to visualize flow within a vessel (i.e. more parallel to direction of flow), and adjust your scale to suit the flow conditions (i.e. higher flow = higher scale, to optimize your image and reduce aliasing).

4. If your images will not be readily available for the surgeon, consider marking the patient to demonstrate the location of the clot:

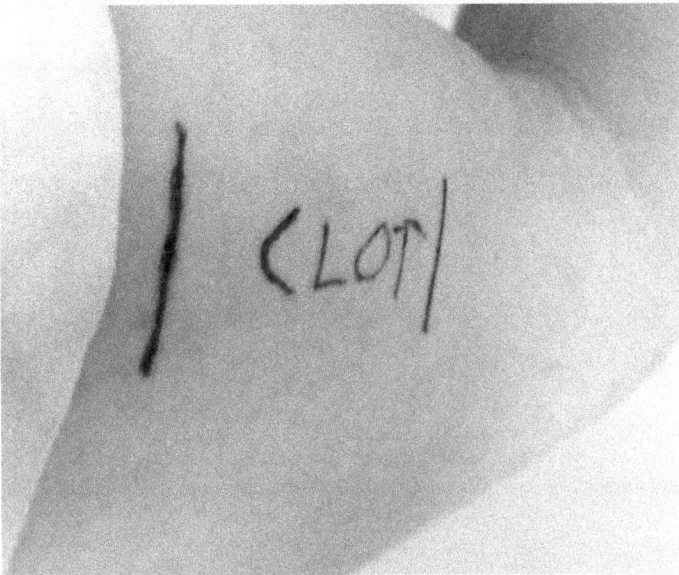

REFERENCES

1. Cook T, Nolting L, Barr C, Hunt P. Diagnostic ultrasonography for peripheral vascular emergencies. Crit Care Clin 2014;30(2):185-206. PMID: 24606773.

2. Rolston DM, Saul T, Wong T, Lewiss RE. Bedside ultrasound diagnosis of acute embolic femoral artery occlusion. J Emerg Med. 2013 Dec;45(6):897-900. PMID: 23988137.

38F with Right-Sided Abdominal Pain

OBJECTIVES

1. Describe the utility and limitations of ultrasound in the diagnosis of ovarian torsion.
2. List the sonographic findings of ovarian torsion.
3. Recognize the implication of a normal computed tomography (CT) scan in ruling out ovarian torsion.

CASE PRESENTATION

A 38-year-old G3P2 woman presents to your ED with right sided abdominal pain with acute worsening of pain. She denies a prior history of similar symptoms. Pain is located on the right lower quadrant (RLQ) of her abdomen, radiating to the right flank. She denies dysuria, hematuria, vaginal discharge, or bleeding. She tells you that her last menstrual period was about six weeks ago, and had a recent positive home pregnancy test. She has not yet had an obstetrics visit for this pregnancy. On physical exam she appears diaphoretic, writhing in pain, and dry heaving. Her abdomen is soft, with exquisite tenderness to palpation over the RLQ and suprapubic region with no palpable masses. There are no overt peritoneal findings on your examination.

VITAL SIGNS

BP	123/60 mmHg
P	90 bpm
RR	20 breaths/min
O2	98% room air
T	36.4°C

DIFFERENTIAL DIAGNOSIS
Appendicitis
Ectopic pregnancy
Nephrolithiasis
Ovarian cyst
Ovarian torsion
Tubo-ovarian abscess

The broad differential diagnosis of acute severe lower abdominal pain in a pregnant patient provides a difficult predicament for the ED provider. The first-line diagnostic imaging modality (computed tomography (CT), magnetic resonance imaging (MRI), or ultrasound) differs depending on which diagnosis is most suspected. The added complication of a first-trimester pregnancy and risks with radiation also affects imaging study selection.

Fortunately, the emergency physician was able to perform point-of-care ultrasound at the patient's bedside to help rule out several of the most likely diagnoses.

POINT-OF-CARE ULTRASOUND was performed which showed the following:

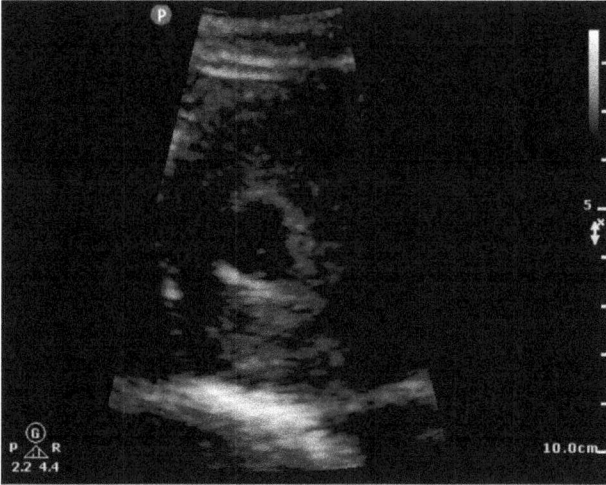

Intrauterine pregnancy identified by intrauterine yolk sac, ruling out ectopic pregnancy

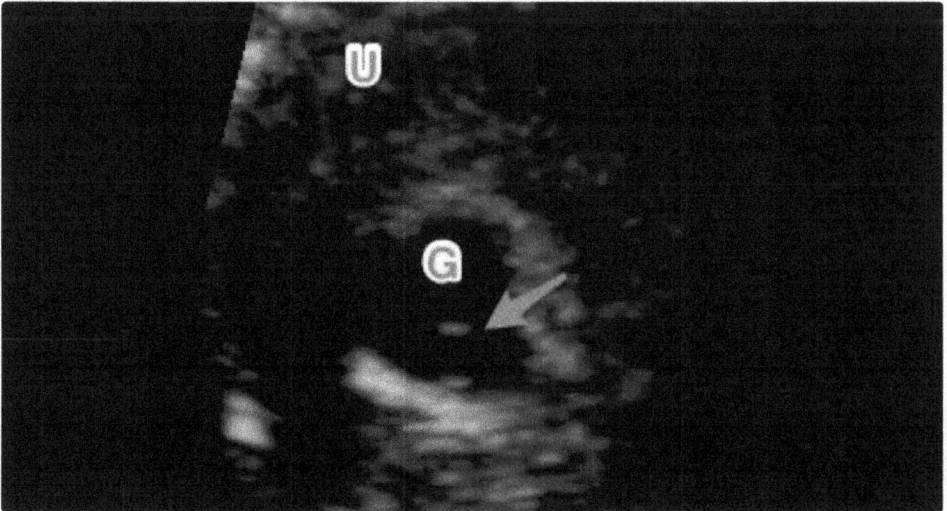

Yolk sac (arrow) appears as a "cheerio" within a gestational sac (G) within the uterus (U)

Figure 11.3

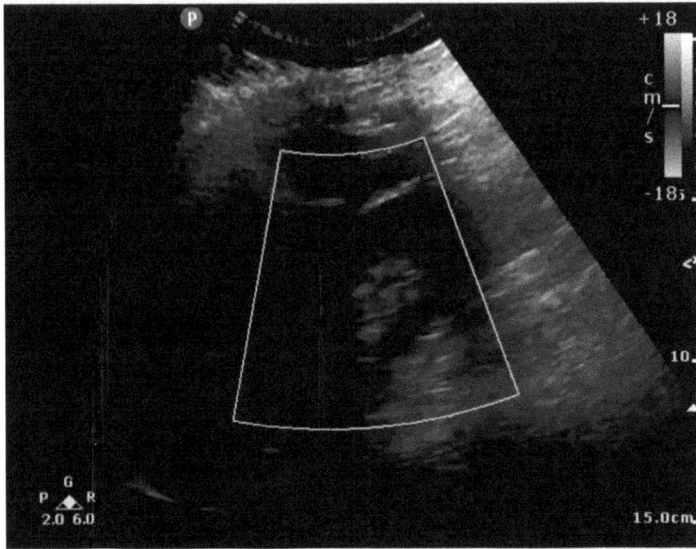

Right kidney with no evidence of hydronephrosis, making renal colic less likely

Figure 11.4

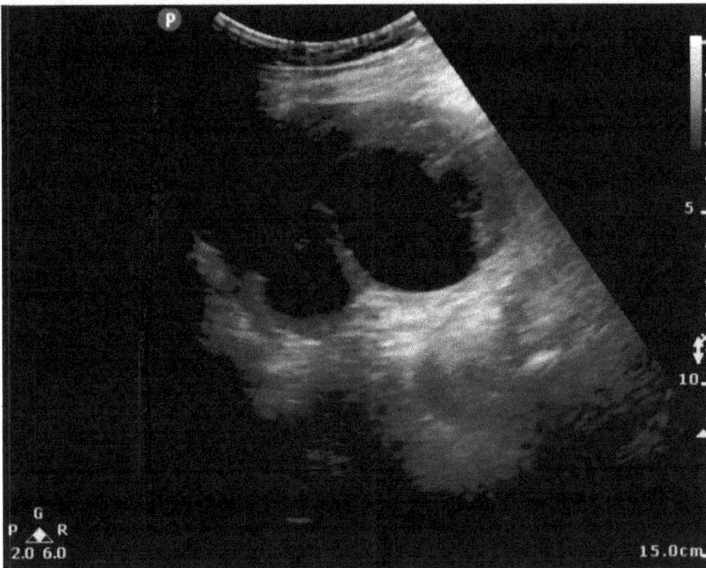

Enlarged right ovary with cystic structures

Figure 11.5

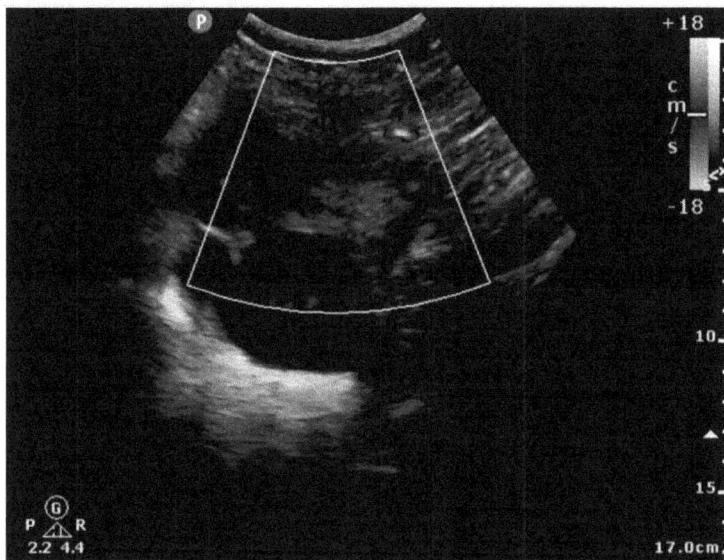

Color Doppler revealing no flow within the ovary but intact flow peripherally

Figure 11.6

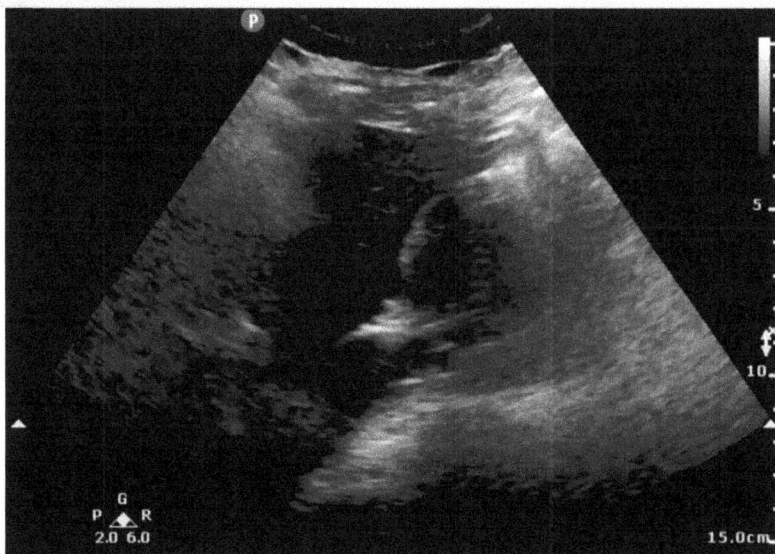

Free fluid in Morison's Pouch, presumably from a ruptured hemorrhagic ovarian cyst

Figure 11.7

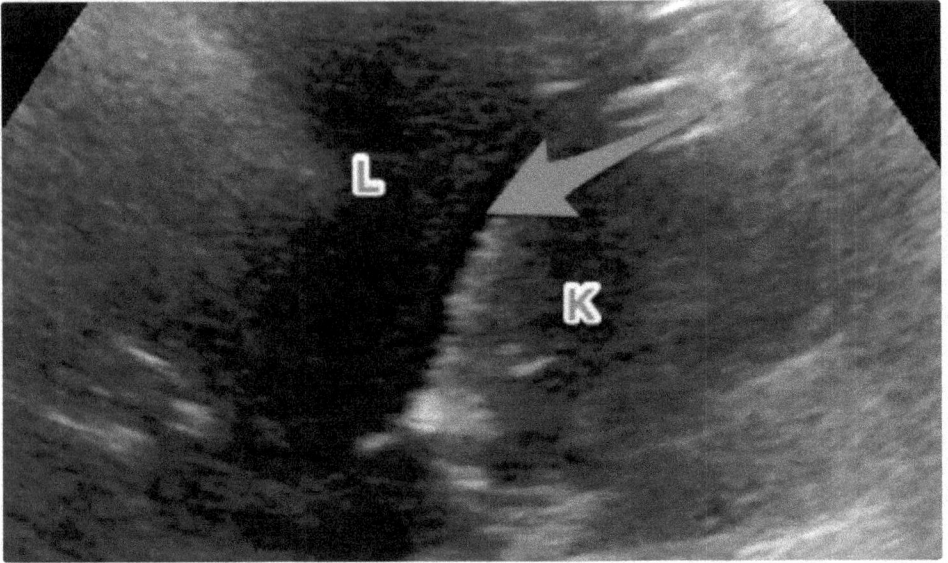

Free fluid (arrow) in Morison's Pouch, between the liver (L) and kidney (K)

The images obtained on the point-of-care ultrasound were able to significantly narrow down the differential diagnosis within minutes, allowing for the ordering of the appropriate radiological studies and consultation for definitive management.

Based these bedside ultrasound findings along with the clinical suspicion for ovarian torsion, gynecology was emergently consulted and a radiology-performed comprehensive ultrasound was ordered.

ULTRASOUND IMAGE QUALITY ASSURANCE

When assessing for ovarian pathology, the use of transvaginal ultrasound is typically required in order to fully evaluate the uterus and adnexae. In this case, however, the right ovary was so enlarged that it could be easily seen transabdominally on ultrasound.

Pelvic ultrasonography for first-trimester pregnancy is considered a core emergency ultrasound application by the American College of Emergency Physicians (ACEP). Ectopic pregnancy should be considered in every woman who presents with abdominal pain or vaginal bleeding with a positive pregnancy test. Emergency physicians can confirm an intrauterine pregnancy (IUP) with 100% specificity when using the criteria of the appearance of a yolk sac, which appears as a "cheerio" (Fig. 11.2), or fetal pole within a gestational sac [1][2]. With a confirmed IUP, the risk of a combined (i.e. heterotopic) pregnancy is extremely rare, with an estimated incidence of 1:4,000-1:8,000 [3], and can essentially be ruled out. A caveat to this is the patient who is undergoing assisted reproductive technology (ART) which increases the incidence of heterotopic pregnancy to an estimated 1:100 [3]!

While ultrasound is the diagnostic imaging modality of choice for ovarian torsion, the diagnosis is confirmed in the operating room. Unfortunately, the ultrasonographic findings of ovarian torsion are variable, representing the spectrum of disease that encompasses torsion. An enlarged (typically greater than 2×3 cm) or cystic ovary with multiple peripheral follicles has been described [4]. The use of color Doppler can be helpful in supporting the diagnosis of ovarian torsion; the absence of flow within the ovary is highly suggestive of ovarian torsion. The added, albeit more advanced, use of spectral Doppler can additionally distinguish between venous and arterial waveforms, and can be used to calculate a Resistive Index (For more information, refer to Case 4). Torsion is highly unlikely if venous flow is present (PPV 94%) [5]. While venous flow to the ovary is the first to be affected, arterial flow, especially peripherally, can still be present [5], as was seen in the images in this patient [Fig. 11.8]. However, it is important to note that the use of color Doppler alone cannot be used to rule out torsion [6].

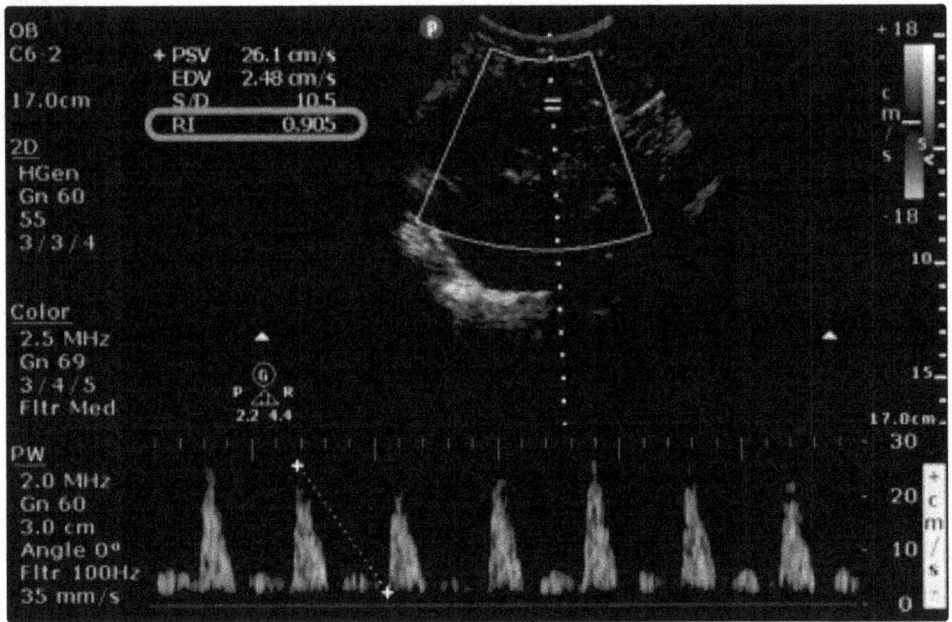

Figure 11.8

Spectral (Pulsed Wave) Doppler reveals arterial flow peripherally with increased resistive index

DISPOSITION AND CASE CONCLUSION

The radiology-performed ultrasound report:

Single live intrauterine pregnancy with an approximate gestational age of 6 weeks 5 days. Right ovary is enlarged, with multiple cysts, with mild high resistance peripheral flow. Patient was exquisitely tender over the right ovary. Appearances are concerning for torsion/detorsion. Clinical correlation is recommended. Left ovary is unremarkable.

Given the prompt consultation, the gynecology team assessed the patient while she was obtaining her comprehensive ultrasound. The patient was consented and taken emergently to the operating room, where right ovarian torsion (twisted 720 degrees) was confirmed, with 200 cc of hemoperitoneum from a ruptured hemorrhagic cyst. The ovary was successfully salvaged, and she remains pregnant with no complications.

Ovarian torsion is a rare but serious surgical emergency that is difficult to diagnose. It is the fifth most common gynecologic emergency with a prevalence of 2.7% [6]. Ovarian torsion is a spectrum of disease that involves twisting of the ovary at its pedicle. Risk factors for torsion are listed in Table 11.1.

RISK FACTORS FOR OVARIAN TORSION
Enlarged ovary
Ovarian cysts/mass
History of pelvic surgery (e.g. tubal ligation)
In-vitro fertilization
Pregnancy

Table 11.1. *Risk Factors for Ovarian Torsion*

The clinical presentation of ovarian torsion is variable and non-specific, but classically involves a sudden-onset of sharp or stabbing unilateral lower quadrant pain with nausea or vomiting [7]. Unfortunately, as these non-specific symptoms overlap with other acute pathologic processes such as renal colic, it is often misdiagnosed. A 15-year review of confirmed cases of ovarian torsion showed high rates of initial misdiagnoses, with torsion considered in less than half of all cases. It is important to maintain a high level of clinical suspicion of torsion, as a timely diagnosis and surgical consultation is necessary to maximize the likelihood of salvaging the ovary. The estimated ovarian salvage rates remain low (approximately 10%) [7].

The most common abnormality seen is an enlarged ovary with or without cysts, which act as a fulcrum from which the ovary can twist at its pedicle. A torsed ovary begins with compromise of venous and lymphatic drainage, leading to an edematous and enlarged ovary. As the disease progresses, arterial flow may be compromised. However, given the dual blood supply to the ovaries (from the ovarian and uterine arteries), it is not uncommon to see arterial flow especially in the periphery, with absence of flow within the ovary itself in cases of ovarian torsion.

Given the non-specific presentation and rare prevalence of ovarian torsion, the use of CT imaging is often used to rule out other acute disease processes when the clinical picture is unclear. A 20-year retrospective review by Moore et al. sought to determine if CT could be used to rule out ovarian torsion. They found that all surgically-confirmed cases of ovarian torsion in the study revealed an abnormal ovary (i.e. enlarged, ovarian cyst, or adnexal mass) on CT [8]. It was concluded that a CT with normal, well-visualized ovaries is sufficient to rule out torsion [8]. However, despite this, if the clinical suspicion is high for ovarian torsion, and bedside ultrasound can be used to expediently rule out other acute pathologies (e.g. renal colic, ectopic pregnancy), a radiology-performed comprehensive ultrasound still remains the diagnostic study of choice.

Ovarian torsion is a rare surgical emergency that is often misdiagnosed and presents with non-specific symptoms that overlap with other acute pathologic diseases. The ability to quickly diagnose the condition and obtain prompt surgical consultation is necessary to maximize ovarian salvage rates.

TAKE-HOME POINTS

1. Ovarian torsion is a rare surgical emergency that presents with non-specific symptoms and requires early diagnosis and surgical consultation to maximize the chance of salvaging the ovary.

2. Ultrasonographic findings of ovarian torsion include an enlarged (greater than 2×3 cm) or cystic ovary, absence of color Doppler flow, or lack of venous flow with spectral Doppler.

3. Point-of-care ultrasound can be used to rule out other acute conditions that present similarly, thus narrowing down your differential diagnosis.

4. While not considered the imaging modality of choice, CT can be used to essentially rule out ovarian torsion, if unremarkable, well-visualized ovaries are seen [8].

REFERENCES

1. Durham B, Lane B, Burbridge L, Balasubramaniam S. Pelvic ultrasound performed by emergency physicians for the detection of ectopic pregnancy in complicated first-trimester pregnancies. Ann Emerg Med. 1997 Mar;29(3): 338-47. PMID: 9055772.

2. Mateer JR, Valley VT, Aiman EJ, Phelan MB, Thoma ME, Kefer MP. Outcome analysis of a protocol including bedside endovaginal sonography in patients at risk for ectopic pregnancy. Ann Emerg Med. 1996 Mar;27(3):283-9. PMID: 8599484.

3. Lambert MJ, Villa M. Gynecologic ultrasound in emergency medicine. Emerg Med Clin North Am. 2004 Aug;22(3):683-96. PMID: 15301846.

4. Ben-Ami M, Perlitz Y, Haddad S. The effectiveness of spectral and color Doppler in predicting ovarian torsion. A prospective study. Eur J Obstet Gynecol Reprod Biol. 2002 Aug 5;104(1):64-6. PMID: 12128265.

5. Albayram F and Hamper UM. Ovarian and adnexal torsion: spectrum of sonographic findings with pathologic correlation. J Ultrasound Med. 2001. Oct;20(10):1083-9. PMID: 11587015.

6. Houry D, Abbott JT. Ovarian torsion: a fifteen-year review. Ann Emerg Med. 2001 Aug;38(2):156-9. PMID: 11468611.

7. Moore C, Meyers AB, Capotasto J, Bokhari J. Prevalence of abnormal CT findings in patients with proven ovarian torsion and a proposed triage schema. Emerg Radiol. 2009 Mar;16(2):115-20. PMID: 18679730.

8. Breyer MJ, Costantino TG. Heterotopic gestation: another possibility for the emergency bedside ultrasonographer to consider. J Emerg Med. 2004 Jan; 26(1):81-4. PMID: 14751482.

55M with Chest Pain

OBJECTIVES

1. Describe the diagnostic utility of point-of-care echocardiography in risk-stratifying patients who present with chest pain.
2. Recognize the significance of echocardiography in identifying regional wall motion abnormalities at the bedside.
3. Name the mnemonic used when identifying regional wall motion abnormalities on the parasternal short axis view.
4. List two caveats that limits the utility of echocardiography in identifying regional wall motion abnormalities.

CASE PRESENTATION

A 55-year-old man walks into your ED with a complaint of left-sided chest pain. He was walking his dog outside 1 hour prior to arrival in the ED when he developed sudden-onset of crushing chest pain. His past medical history includes hypertension and hyperlipidemia, but he denies a prior history of coronary artery disease. He took aspirin and his wife's nitroglycerin without relief. He acknowledges associated shortness of breath. On physical examination, you observe a middle-aged, diaphoretic, and overweight man. His heart sounds are regular without murmurs, and his lungs are clear to auscultation bilaterally. His extremities are warm with no edema.

VITAL SIGNS

BP	115/75 mmHg
P	76 bpm
RR	23 breaths/min
O2	97% room air
T	37.4°C

DIFFERENTIAL DIAGNOSIS

Acute coronary syndrome
Aortic dissection
Pneumothorax
Pulmonary embolism

POINT-OF-CARE ULTRASOUND was performed which showed the following:

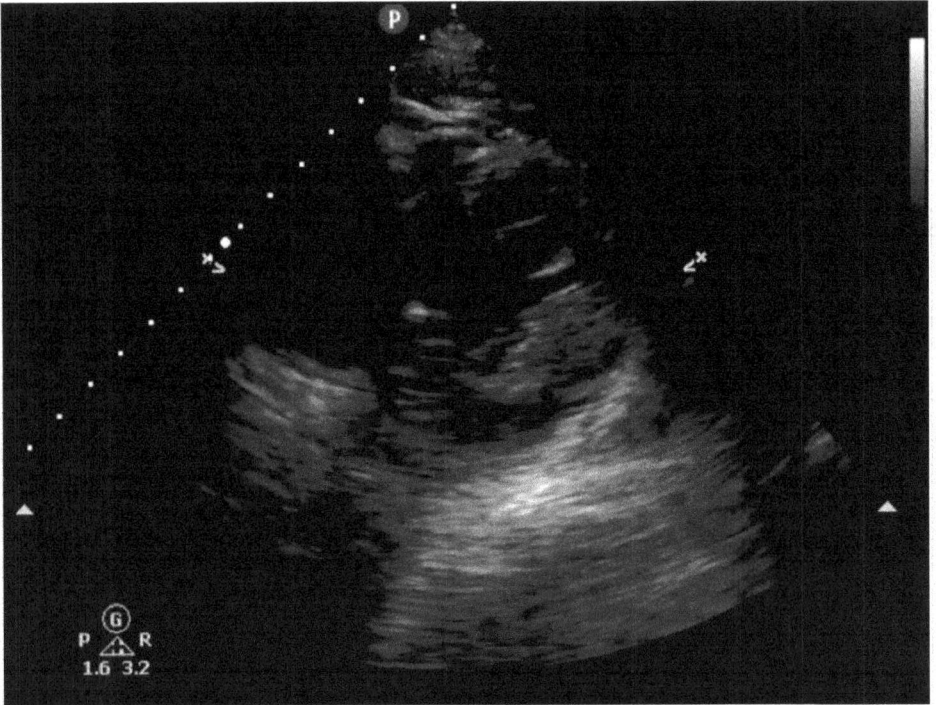

Figure 12.1

Parasternal short axis (PSSA) view revealing hypokinetic septal and anterior segments

Figure 12.2

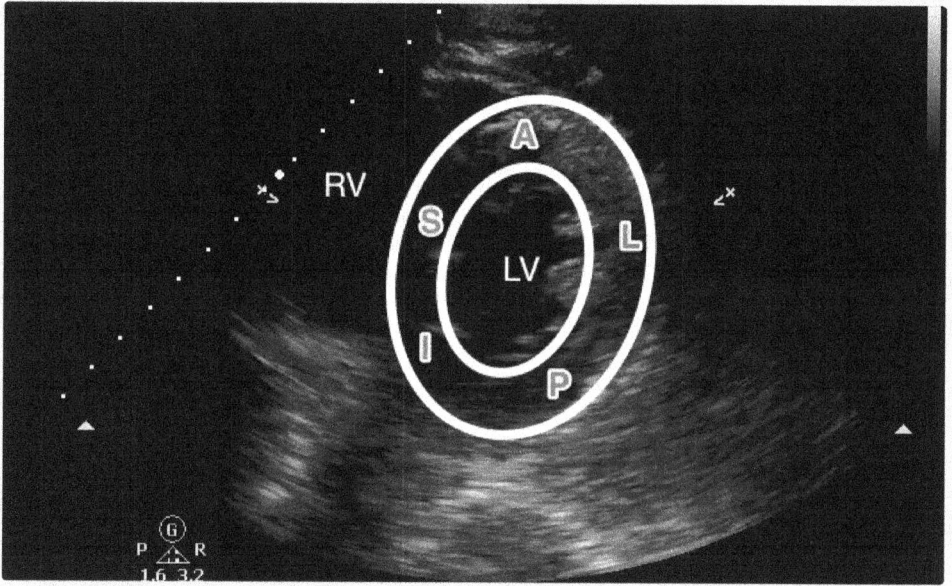

Identification of areas of the left ventricle (LV), "SALPI": Septal (S), Anterior (A), Lateral (L), Posterior (P), Inferior (I). Right ventricle (RV) is also seen.

Figure 12.3

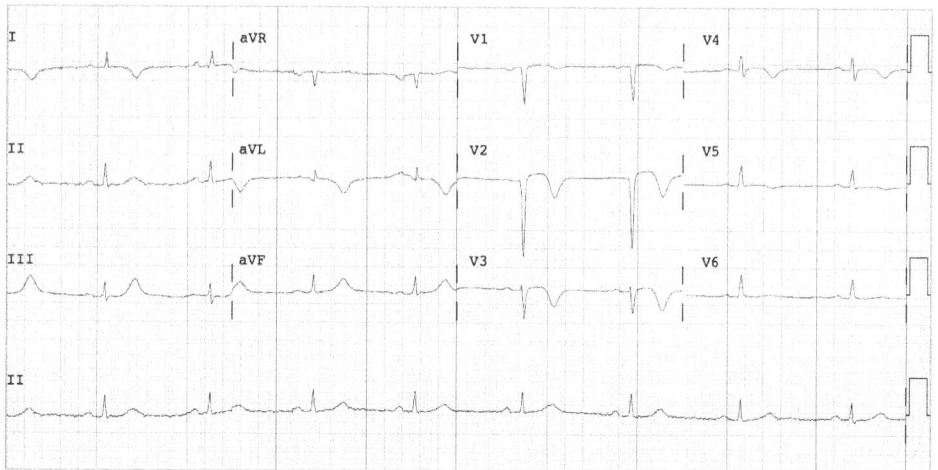

Electrocardiogram (ECG) concerning for anterior ST-elevation myocardial infarction (STEMI)

117

The patient's symptoms along with the ECG (Fig. 12.3) and correlating bedside echo (Fig. 12.1) were concerning for an acute myocardial infarction. The cardiac catheterization lab was thus activated.

ULTRASOUND IMAGE QUALITY ASSURANCE

The ability to identify regional wall motion abnormalities (RWMAs) on echocardiography is considered an advanced but important skill for emergency physicians. For further discussion on proper probe orientation and various cardiac views, please refer to Case 2.

Arguably the most useful view to identify RWMAs is the parasternal short axis view, with the probe marker oriented to the patient's right hip, producing an image that cuts through the left ventricle (LV) in its short axis (Fig. 12.4). Seen on this clip is normal concentric contraction and adequate muscle thickening throughout all regions of the left ventricle.

Figure 12.4

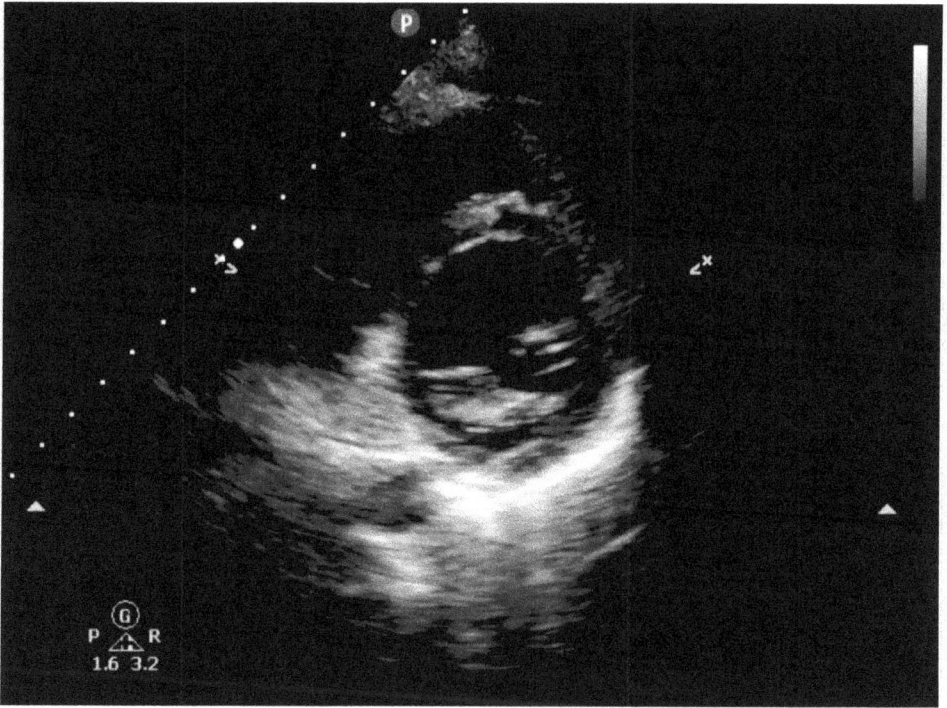

Normal parasternal short axis (PSSA) view of the heart

Using the PSSA view, regions of the left ventricle can be identified using the mnemonic "SALPI" (Fig. 12.2). RWMAs are identified by visualizing areas of hypokinesis or akinesis. More specifically, looking at how well the cardiac muscle thickens during systole is helpful in identifying wall motion abnormalities. Once RWMAs are identified, these can generally be attributed to ischemia of a coronary vessel(s) (Fig. 12.5, Table 12.1). In the images obtained in this case, the septal and anterior portions are hypokinetic correlating to ischemia of the left anterior descending (LAD) artery.

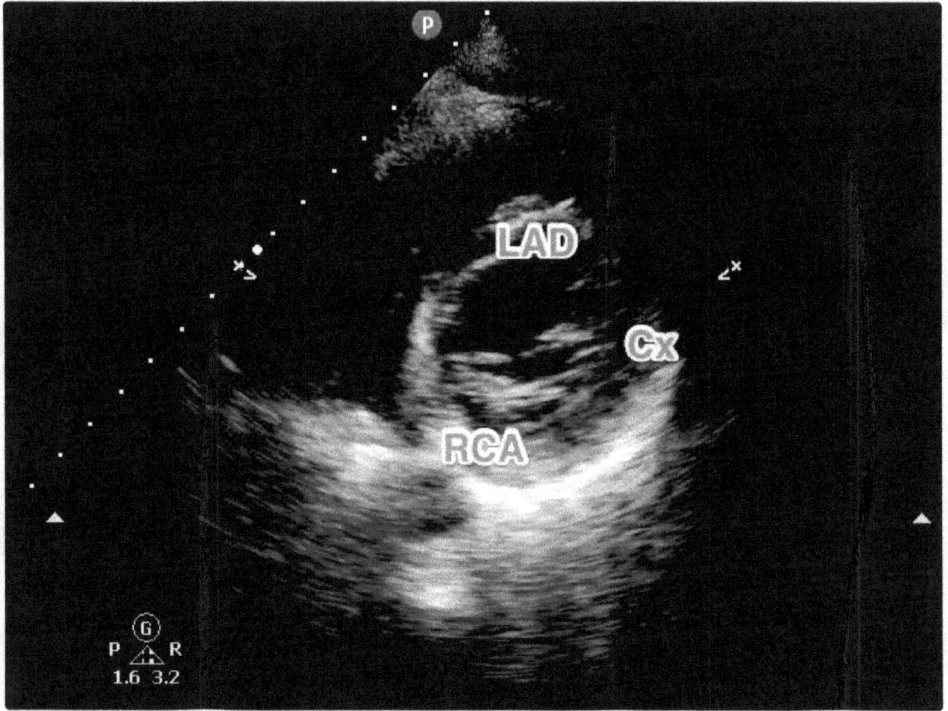

Figure 12.5

Generalized correlation of left ventricular wall regions with coronary vessels; left anterior descending (LAD), circumflex (Cx), and right coronary artery (RCA)

REGION OF LEFT VENTRICLE	CORONARY VESSEL
Septum, Anterior, and Apex	Left anterior descending (LAD)
Lateral	Circumflex (Cx)
Inferior	Right coronary artery (RCA)

Table 12.1. *Correlation of regional wall motion abnormality to ischemia of a coronary vessel.*

DISPOSITION AND CASE CONCLUSION

The patient was emergently taken to the cardiac catheterization lab, where he was found to have a complete acute occlusion of the proximal LAD. His troponin I eventually came back, elevated at 0.16 ng/mL. He underwent a successful thrombectomy and stenting, and was observed in the hospital for 72 hours. He has since been discharged and is doing well!

More than 5 million people present to ED with chest pain [1], and it is important to be able to risk stratify these patients and identify those with acute coronary syndrome (ACS). However, this diagnosis remains a difficult, resource and time-intensive task with a high potential morbidity and mortality.

While the electrocardiogram (ECG) in this case was diagnostic of a STEMI, this is often not the case for patients who present to the ED with acute coronary syndrome. While an ECG is the most widely used screening tool, it is only diagnostic in the minority of cases [2]. In fact, the initial ECG is diagnostic for predicting cardiac events including acute myocardial infarction and/or revascularization in only 40% of patients, while the sensitivity for echocardiogram is much higher at 90% [1]. The reason behind this lies in the concept that ECGs are appropriate for identifying infarction, whereas an echo can identify ischemia without infarction, since necrosis is not needed to cause wall motion abnormalities.

The usefulness of an echocardiogram to identify RWMAs cannot be understated; studies have found that RWMAs are found in 90-100% of patients with a transmural infarction, and 86% of patients with non-Q-wave myocardial infarction [2]. However, the utility of the bedside echocardiogram lies not only in identifying cases of ACS, but also in identifying patients who are at low risk for ACS. A normal echocardiogram performed during active chest pain is a strong predictor of a non-ischemic etiology [3]. Additionally, alternate causes for chest pain, such as cardiac tamponade or a pulmonary embolism, may be evident on the echocardiogram.

Emergency physicians have the unique opportunity to perform a bedside echocardiogram immediately upon a patient's presentation. In the acute setting where "time is muscle", sending a patient to get an echocardiogram by a cardiologist or ultrasound technician may not be a viable option. A study by Kerwin et al. found that after a brief training video, emergency physicians can identify RWMAs with 87% accuracy [4]. The ability to perform a bedside echocardiogram, in conjunction with the clinical scenario and other diagnostic tests, allows emergency physicians to quickly identify patients with a non-diagnostic ECG who may benefit from urgent cath lab activation. It is important to note that RWMAs have been shown to be the first clinically evident sign of acute cardiac ischemia, before ECG and even chest pain [5].

There are caveats to identifying RWMAs on echo; namely patients with prior/old lesions, obtaining adequate cardiac views, and patients with existing significant left-ventricular dysfunction. In these cases, however, patients are at higher risk for ACS and would likely benefit for further investigations.

In summary, in patients at risk for ACS and a non-diagnostic ECG, a bedside echocardiogram performed by the emergency physician can be a useful diagnostic tool that can be used to supplement the clinical scenario.

TAKE-HOME POINTS

1. Bedside echocardiography can be a useful supplemental diagnostic tool to risk-stratify patients who present to the Emergency Department with chest pain.

2. Regional wall motion abnormalities on echocardiography is the earliest clinically evident sign of ischemia and is more sensitive for predicting cardiac events than both ECG changes and onset of chest pain.

3. Caveats to the bedside echocardiogram in identifying regional wall motion abnormalities include prior infarcts and inadequate cardiac views.

REFERENCES

1. Kontos MC, Arrowood JA, Paulsen WH, Nixon JV. Early echocardiography can predict cardiac events in emergency department patients with chest pain. Ann Emerg Med. 1998; 31(5): 550-7. PMID: 9581137.

2. Lee TH, Cook EF, Weisberg M, Sargent RK, Wilson C, Goldman L. Acute chest pain in the emergency room. Identification and examination of low-risk patients. Arch Intern Med. 1985; 145(1): 65-9. PMID: 3970650.

3. Peels CH, Visser CA, Kupper AJ, Visser FC, Roos JP. Usefulness of two-dimensional echocardiography for immediate detection of myocardial ischemia in the emergency room. Am J Cardiol. 1990; 65(11): 687-91. PMID: 2316447.

4. Kerwin C, Tommaso L, Kulstad E. A brief training module improves recognition of echocardiographic wall-motion abnormalities by emergency medicine physicians. Emerg Med Int. 2011; 2011: 483242. PMID: 22046540.

5. Sabia P, Afrookteh A, Touchstone DA, Keller MW, Esquivel L, Kaul S. Value of regional wall motion abnormality in the emergency room diagnosis of acute myocardial infarction. A prospective study using two-dimensional echocardiography. Circulation. 1991; 84(3 Suppl): I85-92. PMID: 1884510.

63M with an Erythematous Abdomen

OBJECTIVES

1. Describe the clinical findings of necrotizing fasciitis and the importance of early diagnosis.
2. Recognize the ultrasonographic findings suggestive of necrotizing fasciitis.
3. Be able to utilize and interpret the LRINEC (Laboratory Risk Indicator for Necrotizing Fasciitis) Score in cases suspicious for possible necrotizing fasciitis.

CASE PRESENTATION

A 63-year-old man with history of diabetes, hypertension, and hyperlipidemia presents with a painful area on his right lower abdomen. He states he noticed pain and redness today, and that it has been worsening over the course of the day. He denies any previous history of similar symptoms and denies trauma. On physical examination, he is a morbidly obese gentleman, in no acute distress. Examination of his abdomen reveals a 10 cm x 12 cm erythematous and tender area on the surface of the right side of his lower abdomen. The area is warm to touch without fluctuance or crepitus. Genitourinary examination is unremarkable.

VITAL SIGNS	
BP	173/82 mmHg
P	111 bpm
RR	23 breaths/min
O2	97% room air
T	37.9°C

DIFFERENTIAL DIAGNOSIS

Abscess
Cellulitis
Necrotizing Fasciitis

LABORATORY INVESTIGATIONS

- Total White Blood Cell count: 18 x mm3

- C-Reactive Protein: 240 mg/L

- Hemoglobin: 14.3 g/dL

- Sodium: 139 mmol/L

- Creatinine: 119 umol/L (or 1.35 mg/dL)

- Glucose: 12 mmol/L (or 216 mg/dL)

- Lactate: 4.1 mmol/L

POINT-OF-CARE ULTRASOUND was performed which showed the following:

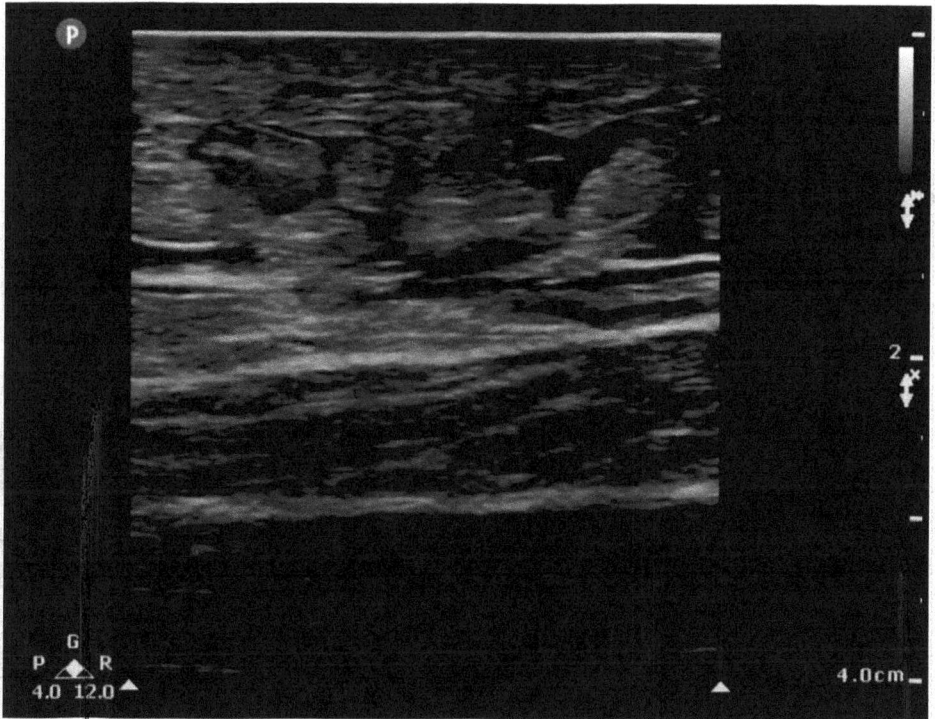

Figure 13.1

Cobblestoning of subcutaneous soft tissue with fluid in the deeper fascial plane.

Figure 13.2

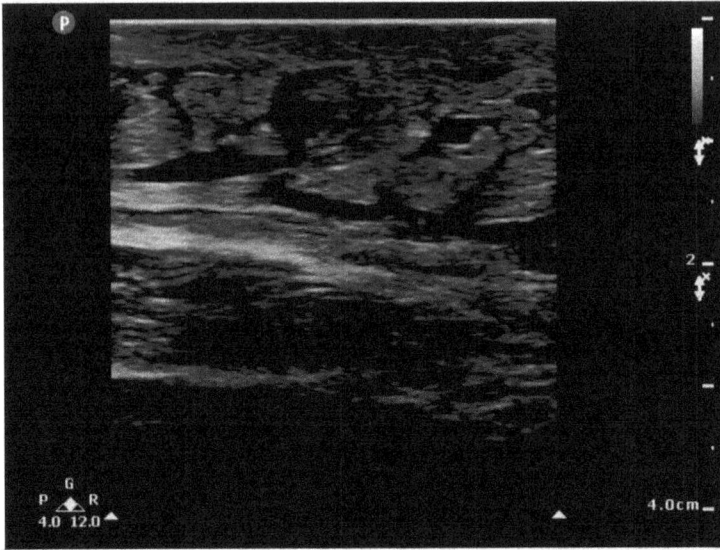

Cobblestoning of subcutaneous soft tissue with fluid in the deeper fascial plane.

Figure 13.3

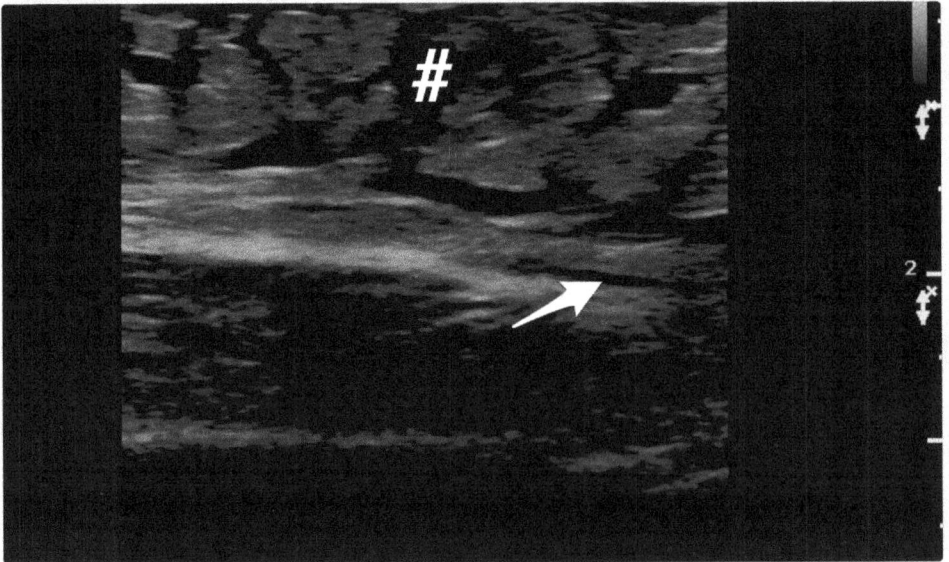

Cobblestoning of the subcutaneous tissue (#) and fluid in the deep fascial plane (arrow) is seen.

ULTRASOUND IMAGE QUALITY ASSURANCE

The ultrasound images were obtained using the high-frequency linear probe, which is beneficial when attempting to visualize superficial structures within a few centimeters from the surface. The images reveal cobblestoning of the subcutaneous tissue, a non-specific finding that can be seen with cellulitis [Fig. 13.1, Fig. 13.2]. Of note, the subcutaneous tissue is uniformly thickened; a comparison of a normal area (e.g. a contralateral limb) can be visualized to confirm abnormal thickening. Deep to the subcutaneous layer is the deep fascial plane, where abnormal fluid is seen in this case [Fig. 13.3]. These findings can be seen with necrotizing fasciitis. As the disease progresses, abnormal air, visualized as "dirty shadowing" on ultrasound, may be seen in late and more severe cases.

DISPOSITION AND CASE CONCLUSION

Given the concerning history and physical examination along with the point-of-care ultrasound concerning for necrotizing fasciitis, empiric antibiotics (IV vancomycin and piperacillin/tazobactam) were given, and surgery was consulted.

The patient was taken to the operating room where a wash out and debridement was performed with a confirmed diagnosis of necrotizing fasciitis. The patient was monitored in the intensive care unit post-operatively and has since been discharged and is doing well.

Background on Necrotizing Fasciitis

Necrotizing fasciitis is a rare (with an incidence of 4.3 infections per 100,000 in the United States), but severe soft tissue infection [1,2]. The most severe form of soft tissue infections, necrotizing fasciitis is a rapidly progressing infection of the subcutaneous tissue and fascia that is potentially limb and life threatening, with a mortality rate of up to 76% [2,3]. Bacterial enzymes cause tissue necrosis, leading to fluid that can be visualized in the deep fascial layer. The typical bacterial pathogens involved in necrotizing fasciitis include staphylococci, streptococci, and anaerobes, and antibiotic coverage should provide broad coverage for these organisms [4]. Definitive management requires operative debridement and potential fasciotomy.

The classic physical examination findings of necrotizing fasciitis, including a rapidly progressing area of erythema with ill-defined borders, are often indistinguishable from other soft tissue infections including cellulitis and abscess, especially early in the disease process. Thus, a high index of clinical suspicion is required in the Emergency Department [2]. While physical exam findings including blistering, hemorrhagic bullae, and crepitus can increase the suspicion of necrotizing fasciitis, these are often late findings seen only in severe and progressed cases [2]. While necrotizing fasciitis is considered a clinical diagnosis, there may be some utility for laboratory tests and point-of-care ultrasound to aid in risk-stratifying equivocal cases.

LRINEC Score

The LRINEC (Laboratory Risk Indicator for Necrotizing Fasciitis) score utilizes 6 common laboratory tests to risk stratify patients with concern for possible necrotizing fasciitis (Table 1) [3]. A score of ≥6 should raise your suspicion of the diagnosis, while a score of ≥8 is strongly predictive of necrotizing fasciitis [3]. In this case, the LRINEC score is 6, which increases the suspicion of necrotizing fasciitis.

Ultrasound Findings for Necrotizing Fasciitis

Ultrasound can also be used to identify patients with necrotizing fasciitis. While CT and MRI have been the more traditionally used imaging modalities, they are time consuming, costly, and delay the time to definitive operative management. The ultrasonographic findings of necrotizing fasciitis include diffuse thickening of the subcutaneous tissue when compared to the contralateral side or limb, and

LAB, UNITS	SCORE
C-REACTIVE PROTEIN, mg/L	
< 150	0
≥ 150	4
WHITE CELL COUNT, per mm3	
< 15	0
15 - 25	1
> 25	2
HEMOGLOBIN, g/dL	
> 13.5	0
11 - 13.5	1
< 11	2
SODIUM, mmol/L	
≥ 135	0
< 135	2
CREATININE	
≤ 141 mmol/L or 1.6 mg/dL	0
> 141 mmol/L or 1.6 mg/dL	2
GLUCOSE	
≤ 10 mmol/L or 180 mg/dL	0
> 10 mmol/L or 180 mg/dL	1

Table 13.1. Laboratory Risk Indicator for Necrotizing Fasciitis (LRINEC) Score.

LRINEC Score > 6 should raise suspicion of necrotizing fasciitis. Score > 8 is strongly predictive of necrotizing fasciitis. (Modified from Wong et al.)

a layer of fluid seen more than 4 mm deep along the deep fascial layer [1]. Using these criteria, ultrasound has been shown to be 88.2% sensitive, 93.3% specific, and 91.9% accurate [1]. As the disease progresses, air within the fascial layer, seen as "dirty shadowing" may be seen. A useful mnemonic has been described in the literature as the STAFF exam (Subcutaneous Thickening, Air, and Fascial Fluid) [2].

Necrotizing fasciitis remains a clinical diagnosis, and concern for the disease requires prompt surgical consultation. While laboratory tests (LRINEC score) and ultrasound are beneficial and can aid in the risk stratification and diagnosis of cases, they should not be used solely to rule out the disease.

TAKE-HOME POINTS

1. Necrotizing fasciitis is a rare but potentially limb and life threatening infection, requiring a high index of clinical suspicion.

2. While necrotizing fasciitis is a clinical diagnosis, the LRINEC score and point-of-care ultrasound can aid in the risk-stratification and early diagnosis of the disease.

3. Ultrasonographic findings suggestive of necrotizing fasciitis include:

    • Fascial and subcutaneous thickening

    • Fluid in the deep fascial layer

    • Subcutaneous air

REFERENCES

1. Yen Z, Wang H, Ma H, Chen S, Chen W. Ultrasonographic screening of clinically-suspected necrotizing fasciitis. Acad Emerg Med. 2002;9(12): 1448-1451. PMID: 12460854.

2. Castleberg E, Jenson N, Dinh V. Diagnosis of necrotizing faciitis with bedside ultrasound: the STAFF Exam. West J Emerg Med. 2014;15(1):111-113. PMID: 24578776.

3. Wong C, Khin L, Heng K, Tan K, Low C. The LRINEC (Laboratory Risk Indicator for Necrotizing Fasciitis) score: a tool for distinguishing necrotizing fasciitis from other soft tissue infections. Crit Care Med. 2004;32(7):1535-1541. PMID: 15241098.

4. Green R, Dafoe D, Raffin T. Necrotizing fasciitis. Chest. 1996;110(1):219-229. PMID: 8681631.

Appendix